The AIDS Benefits Handbook

Thomas P. McCormack

THE AIDS BENEFITS HANDBOOK

Everything You Need to Know to Get Social Security, Welfare, Medicaid, Medicare, Food Stamps, Housing, Drugs, and Other Benefits

Yale University Press   New Haven and London

Designed by Richard Hendel.
Set in Times Roman type by
The Composing Room of Michigan, Inc.
Printed in the United States of America by
Vail-Ballou Press, Binghamton, N.Y.

The paper in this book meets the guidelines for
permanence and durability of the Committee on
Production Guidelines for Book Longevity of the
Council on Library Resources.

10 9 8 7 6 5 4 3 2 1

Library of Congress
Cataloging-in-Publication Data
McCormack, Thomas P., 1944–
    The AIDS benefits handbook : everything
you need to know to get social security,
welfare, medicaid, medicare, food stamps,
housing, drugs, and other benefits / Thomas P.
McCormack.
        p.   cm.
    Includes bibliographical references.
    ISBN 0-300-04736-3 (alk. paper) —
ISBN 0-300-04721-5 (pbk. : alk. paper)
    1. AIDS (Disease) —Patients—Services
for—United States—handbooks, manuals,
etc.   2. Social security—United States—
Handbooks, manuals, etc.   I. Title.
RC607.A26M38   1990   89-70591
362.1'9697'9200973—dc20   CIP

This book is dedicated to the

memory of Katherine Beaumont,

who never let me forget that

"within broad federal regulations,

each state administers its own *program."*

Contents

Appendices

Preface

By early 1990, more than 100,000 Americans have been diagnosed as having Acquired Immune Deficiency Syndrome (AIDS), and even more suffer from the disabling conditions of AIDS-Related Complex (ARC). Indeed, the federal Centers for Disease Control (CDC) in Atlanta estimates that there will be 80,000 additional AIDS cases by 1992, and that 170,000 will then be under active treatment for AIDS, with the cumulative total cases rising to 450,000 by 1993. However, these people and their advocates generally have virtually no personal knowledge of public benefit programs or their eligibility rules—unlike the *traditional* poor, disabled, and elderly who have long had the advocacy support with which to access benefits.

This handbook hopes to remedy this knowledge deficiency among persons with AIDS (PWAs) and their advocates by offering this brief encyclopedia of income, health, and housing programs for the disabled. It grew out of training materials prepared by the author for fellow PWA entitlements advocates at the Whitman-Walker Clinic, a Washington, D.C., PWA health and social service organization. The project was further motivated by the lack of any meaningful benefits advocacy staff, programs, or training manuals at the major AIDS-related organizations in Washington, D.C.—the AIDS Action Council, the National AIDS Network, and the National Association of People with AIDS. The staff of all three groups have been interested in this project at its various stages of development.

Many public programs help those citizens who are disabled, but no single program meets all needs. This handbook is designed to help persons with human immunodeficiency virus (HIV) disease and their advocates to select and use those public programs which can best meet their needs. The writer sincerely hopes that it will be widely used and that increasing numbers of people with HIV disease will receive the full range of benefits to which they are entitled.

The author earnestly invites comments, corrections and additional information from readers interested in the field. Please write to him at P.O. Box 27591, Washington, D.C. 20038.

Acknowledgments

No one can complete the often interminable research for a book of this complexity without feeling compelled to thank those many advisors and informants who made it possible. Only the writer really knows his debts—no matter how routine acknowledgments listings may seem to readers.

Even after nearly twenty years in and around the wondrously complex eligibility system, I would have been hopelessly at sea without the generous and expert support of those who so kindly led me through the jungles of our American domestic assistance programs. My gratitude is immense.

I particularly wish to thank those whose help I have inadvertently omitted to mention; in a project this size such an oversight was perhaps inevitable; it is still lamentable.

I owe thanks to: Ron Benschotter of the AIDS Action Council; Audrey Doughty and Patrick James of AIDS Benefits Counselors, fellow mapmakers in the eligibility quest; Marcia Lipetz of the AIDS Foundation of Chicago; George Gaberlavage, Marilyn Moon, and Doris Reeves-Lipscomb of the American Association of Retired Persons; John Covell of Yale University Press, for many helpful suggestions and direction; Tony Borden of *American Lawyer;* Clint Hockenberry of the AIDS Legal Referral Panel; Marc Scheuppert of Boston AIDS Action; Penelope Ashcroft, Emmet Dye, and Bob Shelbourne of the Family Support Administration, HHS; Ann Milano of the Gay Men's Health Crisis; Mike Fiori, Dick Hall, Jack Luehrs, Gary Martin, Mike McDaniel, Bob McKelney, Lou Shiro, Joyce Stokes, Bob Tomlinson, and Bob Wardwell of the Health Care Financing Administration; Charles Hofstetter and Rick Schulman of the Health Resources and Services Administration; Wendy Schiller of H.E.R.O.; Edward Whipple of the Department of Housing and Urban Development; Ron Gardner of the Houston AIDS Foundation; Walter Bledsoe of the Department of Veterans Affairs; Stephen Beck of the Design Industry Foundation for AIDS; Mr. Marion Shumaker of the Disabled American Veterans; Ms. Pat Rusche of the D.C. Disability Determination Division; Mary Patrick, Ann Gariazo, and Pat Hagen of the Food and Nutrition Service; Frances Goldin and Sydelle Kramer for support, advocacy, and encouragement; Dan Dever and Steve Westphall of the Howard Brown Memorial Clinic; Liz Donahue and

Debra Lipson of the Intergovernmental Health Policy Project; Miguel Gomez of La Raza; Bill Wyland of the Legal Assistance Foundation of Chicago; Michael Schuster and Ayn Crawley of Legal Counsel for the Elderly; Robert Gillett of Legal Services of Southeastern Michigan; Larry Ellis and Robert Thewes of Lifelink; Ms. Lee Carty of the Mental Health Law Project, who is editing a parallel manual for the homeless; Jim Holm, Peter Lee, and Phil Pelino of the National AIDS Network; Bob Hoyt of the National Association for Home Care; Toni Young of the National Association of People With AIDS; Ben Schatz of National Gay Rights Advocates; Sarah Anders and Bruce Fried of the National Health Care Campaign; Michael Dowell, Roger Schwartz, and Judith Waxman of the National Health Law Project; Patti Mellely, formerly with the National Housing Law Project; Kurt Decker of National Protection and Advocacy Systems; Barbara Jameson of the National Residential Care Facilities Association; Eileen Sweeney of the National Senior Citizens' Law Center; Keith Snyder of the National Veterans' Legal Services Project; Ms. Pat Dillion of the Philadelphia AIDS Task Force; Douglas Smith of Physicians' Disability Services; Randy Shilts of the *San Francisco Chronicle;* Diane Blackman, Jennie Cargill, Bob Lorfick, Elsa Ponce, and Dave Smith of the Social Security Administration; Lori Kessler of the South Florida AIDS Network; Sharon Daley of the U.S. Catholic Conference; Betty Ahearn, Nelson Miranda, Carol Rowan, and Mary Sielers of the Veterans' Medical Center in Washington, D.C.; Tom Sherwood of the Vietnam Veterans of America; Jeff Kirsch and Phyllis Torda of the Villers Foundation; and Susan Denise, Ruth Eisenberg, Rusty Lynn, Gail Messier, and Dinah Wiley of the Whitman-Walker Clinic.

The Entitlements Volunteers at the Whitman-Walker Clinic have been my fellow-guides in the PWA benefits maze; we've learned much working together.

I've relied upon Joe James, for his cheerful and accommodating accuracy and patience in preparing and revising a manuscript that escalated in its complexity and length over more than two years, and the many, many people with AIDS, with whom I've struggled and learned, and for whom this book is written.

Introduction

How to Use This Book to Use the Welfare System

This is a book about how to get on welfare. The program-by-program over-views, the summaries of the rules, and the appendices on the most important state-by-state variations just scratch the surface of the often convoluted and widely varying programs available to PWAs and their advocates.

In order to make choices about these programs and, ideally, to secure cover-age by them, readers will find some intelligent review necessary. Given the number of programs, the state variations, and the enormous mass of eligibility rules, such a review is a daunting task. But the stark reality we confront in seeking income and health care for PWAs is that there *is* no alternative to grap-pling with the current system—difficult, frustrating, and enormously intim-idating though it may be. Many college educated, middle class, disabled people and activists become angry, frustrated, contemptuous, and disparaging of the system when they first become aware of its complexities, variations, and te-dious bureaucratic procedures. They dismiss it, and they refuse to engage its workings practically, because they see it as such a hopeless, unworkable mess. Yet millions of grade school-educated welfare mothers and destitute aged and disabled persons negotiate the welfare system's pitfalls with much success each and every month. And if this is so, how much more mastery can be achieved through the patient labors of those of us blessed with more resources?

There is no simple, brief, magical way to learn this welfare system; as the saying goes, "no pain, no gain." Nonetheless, this handbook makes every effort to streamline the road we must travel to work within the American bene-fits system. For a quick overview of the major programs, see the table on these pages.

The Programs

The central programs for newly disabled persons such as PWAs are Social Security Disability Insurance (SSDI), Supplemental Security Income (SSI),

Major Benefits Programs

Aid to Families with Dependent Children (AFDC) is a federal-state program making welfare payments to low-income families with children which include a single, unemployed, or incapacitated parent. In 1988 nearly 11 million recipients received $16.8 billion in assistance through local welfare offices.

AZT Drug Assistance is a federally financed, state-administered program which subsidizes the purchase of AZT (Retrovir) and two other AIDS-related drugs for low-income HIV-infected persons without other drug coverage. In 1989, 6,500 persons received $20 million worth of AZT and other drugs with federal funds through state and local health and welfare agencies.

Emergency Assistance (EA) is a federal-state welfare program which makes one-time emergency grants to or on behalf of low-income families with children facing financial or other crises. These services are provided by local welfare offices and some shelters. In 1988, 540,000 families with children received $230 million in emergency assistance. Many states also provided these services to needy disabled and aged people.

The **Food Stamp (FS)** program is a federally financed, state-run welfare program for all kinds of low-income persons. In 1988, 18.7 million persons received $12.69 billion worth of Food Stamps through local welfare offices.

General Assistance (GA) is a state-local welfare program offered by most states to low-income persons who are not covered by the federal AFDC and SSI assistance programs. In 1988, 1,115,000 persons received payments. General Assistance payments are made by local welfare offices.

General Medical Assistance is a state-local program to finance medical care for low-income persons who are not covered by the federal Medicaid program. In 1982, an estimated $15 billion worth of medical care was provided to these persons through state and local welfare offices, health departments, and public clinics and hospitals.

The **Hill-Burton** program provides federal grants and loans to hospitals and other health facilities for construction, renovation, and expansion. In exchange, thousands of beneficiary facilities must (1) give free or reduced-fee medical care to low-income persons and (2) permanently provide health care access services to all who seek them. In 1982, American hospitals provided indigents with $9.5 billion worth of free care, through Hill-Burton and other uncompensated care programs.

Low Income Home Energy Assistance (LIHEA) is a federally financed, state-run program to subsidize the heating, air conditioning, and home weatherization costs of low-income households, particularly those of the aged and disabled. In 1988, $1.4 billion in energy costs were covered.

Medicaid is a federal-state program to finance medical care for the low-income aged, the blind, the disabled, and families and children. In 1987, 24 million persons received $49.5 billion worth of medical care through state and local welfare agencies.

Medicare is a federal health insurance program covering most medical expenses of aged and disabled Social Security recipients. In 1987, 33 million persons were covered, at a cost of $130 billion, through the Social Security Administration (SSA).

The **Social Services Block Grant** program, formerly known as Title XX, is a federally financed, staterun program to provide social services such as counseling, home chore aid, transportation, recreation, job training, rehabilitation, meal programs, and other casework support to low-income persons, especially the aged, the disabled, and families and children. In 1988, federal funds purchased $2.7 billion in services through local welfare offices. This was supplemented by several times that amount in additional state and local appropriations.

Social Security Disability Insurance (SSDI) is a federal program paying income benefits, based on lifetime earnings records, to disabled workers and their families. In 1987, 2.8 million disabled workers received $16.88 billion in payments through local offices of the Social Security Administration (SSA).

Supplemental Security Income (SSI) is a federal welfare program making payments to low-income aged, blind, and disabled persons. In 1987, nearly 5 million persons received about $11 billion in SSI payments from the Social Security Administration (SSA).

State Supplementary Payments (SSPs) are state welfare programs to guarantee and provide income support *above the basic federal SSI level* to low-income aged, blind, and disabled persons. As of early 1989, about 1.5 million disabled persons received SSPs through the Social Security Administration (SSA). (Several hundred thousand other poor disabled people received SSPs through state and local welfare offices.)

The **Temporary Emergency Food Assistance (TEFA)** program distributes surplus stored federal food to low-income persons. In 1988, approximately 15 million persons received free food through local welfare offices, churches, charity groups, and food banks.

The **Department of Veterans Affairs (VA)** is a federal agency providing income support and medical care to disabled veterans of military services, some other veterans, and their families. In 1988, 3.6 million persons received $11.02 billion in VA payments and 3.7 million received $16.3 billion worth of free VA medical care.

AZT Assistance, and Medicaid. The first two are administered by the federal government's Social Security Administration (SSA), while Medicaid is a state-run assistance program; so are the vital but less often used General Assistance (GA), Aid to Families with Dependent Children (AFDC), Emergency Assistance (EA), and Food Stamp (FS) programs. Some veterans can also qualify for important help from the Department of Veterans Affairs (VA) income and health programs. Less often used, but sometimes helpful to PWAs, are the Medicare, Energy Assistance, housing, and mental health programs. Finally, there are several programs of real potential for aiding PWAs, but which are far less well known to the AIDS advocacy community and therefore not used nearly to their potential: the Hill-Burton, state or local indigent medical assistance, and private charity programs available in many hospitals; State Supplementary Payment (SSP) programs to finance PWA group housing in "board and care homes"; and state-run drug (and even health insurance) subsidy programs. This manual reviews all of these and tries to point out their applicability for PWAs.

Dealing with the Welfare Office

Welfare offices (which are, curiously enough, still called just that by both their employees and clients, even though government agencies persist in using euphemisms such as "social services" or "human services" departments), Social

Security district offices and VA Medical and Outreach Centers can be intimidating places. Waits are long and often unpleasant; moreover, one must rub shoulders with the most afflicted members of society. Workers are often rushed and overworked. Bureaucratic jargon, application forms, and notices to applicants can be well-nigh incomprehensible.

Nonetheless, some basic pointers for dealing with offices in all of these programs can be of significant help. First, *always telephone ahead to find out whether an "appointment" to apply is necessary.* In most SSA offices and many welfare offices, it is; in this case the date of the telephone inquiry, rather than the "appointment" date, can be used as the effective application date. Arriving to apply *without* checking about the need for an advance appointment—except in the most leisurely welfare offices—could result in a gruesome wait of several hours, or in not being seen at all.

All this leads to the need to *apply without delay* for all programs, because waiting for a convenient day to do so or to gather the many necessary documents *inevitably causes loss of or delays in benefits.* Unfortunately, delays in applying are quite common in PWA cases, as a result not only of confusion and lack of guidance, but also of the lassitude and depression many PWAs experience. More insidious, however, is the nearly universal compulsion of so many PWAs and their advocates to put off applying while gathering documents—in each case, this can result in the loss of hundreds of dollars in benefits and the potential noncoverage of thousands in medical bills. Advocates need to work a lot harder to prevent delay and file timely applications.

Making Your Case

Welfare eligibility caseworkers *thrive* on documentation and verifications to support application packages. The more thoroughly, the more quickly, the more unprotestingly, the more *imaginatively,* an applicant or advocate meets these requirements (see appendix E), the more likely the case is to be processed quickly and helpfully—or even to be approved at all, in the case of borderline cases. The key point to remember is that workers *hate* to have open, pending, as-yet-undocumented files on their desks—they want to clear their overloaded "pending" baskets. A worker pleased with a timely, responsive applicant will often take the time to explain ways to increase benefits or to describe unfamiliar programs. Be imaginative: if you can't get a typewritten, formal doctor's letter, have the doctor write a note by hand while you wait, and then submit *that;* if you don't have a lease or utility bills in your own name, get a note from your landlord or roommate; if you're homeless, get notes from social workers or shelters verifying that you at least move about within the jurisdiction; show envelopes sent to you in the mail to prove residency; present old passports, driver's licenses, or military forms to show your age and place of birth. Remember, get a note to prove *everything* on your application, even if you have to dictate one to the person you ask to write it.

It's best to deal with eligibility workers *in person;* not only will they remember you more clearly then, and ideally give more timely attention to your case, but this may be the only realistic way to contact them because welfare and Social Security office telephone lines are often jammed. (In fact, SSA encourages the mailing or telephoning of applications with its nationwide toll-free number: 1-800-234-5772. Avoid this whenever possible—apply *in person.*) *Never* send an original document through the mail to an eligibility worker (these are often lost during or after transit) and *never* part with your only copy of any document or verification note—you will need it again when the worker loses it, or when you apply for some other program. Have the worker photocopy your forms and papers while you wait.

Welfare and Social Security offices are crowded and overwhelmed on the first few days of each month (by people who didn't get their checks, Food Stamps, or Medicaid card) and for the last few days of the month (by people who have used up their checks and Food Stamps and want more). Moreover, Mondays and Fridays are also bad days to apply or discuss your case, because many workers take these days off and because many applicants and recipients have "crises" on these days too. The best times to apply are therefore mid-week and mid-month.

Social Workers vs. Eligibility Workers

Most laymen, PWAs, and even experienced AIDS volunteers assume that "social workers" handle benefits eligibility; unfortunately, this is usually not so, and this misunderstanding can sometimes result in eligibility problems. All welfare departments are actually divided into *two* separate, parallel bureaucracies: "eligibility" and "services." "Services" employees are social workers and usually hold graduate degrees and accreditation in social work (for example, M.S.W., L.C.S.W., or A.C.S.W.). They worry about clients' psychological state, home life, social support, and medical care problems. Those dealing with families and children have well-defined roles in handling child or spouse abuse, and in arranging foster care for children, adoptions, marital counseling, vocational assessment, and other services. Today's social workers—both those who work in the "service" part of welfare offices and their counterparts in hospitals—are anything but stereotypical prim spinsters; their present roles include services referral coordinator, mental health and family therapist, and overall case manager. *All* have a general knowledge of benefits eligibility (although this is not emphasized in their graduate schools or even in their employee training); *most* feel confident in advising about entitlements; but *very few have a specialized, detailed knowledge of programs' eligibility.* Social workers are *not* eligibility workers!

Who, then, is responsible for and who determines eligibility? *Eligibility workers* (also known by such titles as eligibility technicians, caseworkers, case aides, social service representatives, claims representatives, and benefits specialists) *determine eligibility.* These are the folks who staff the *other* half of the welfare office (although you won't find any of them on hospital social work staffs). They almost always specialize—as AFDC workers, GA workers, Medicaid-only workers, nursing home Medicaid workers, Food Stamp workers, or Social Security/SSI claims representatives—and they *generally* are knowledgeable only about the rules of the program to which they are assigned (unless they are supervisors with wide experience, or are unusually adept intellectually). In most areas, eligibility workers are, and are treated as, glorified, nonprofessional clerks. They are most often workers with high-school-level educations, although in some urban and suburban offices inroads have been made by the college educated.

What all this means is that those who *can* articulately explain the system and propose creative "solutions" for difficult cases are those eligibility supervisors and administrators who have been around the local system for a while and who have the insight to do so with confidence. Those advocating on behalf of PWAs need to identify and meet with these people to get a local program-by-program education, and then secure their intervention when complex problem cases arise.

Social Workers and Eligibility in Hospitals

Hospitals present something of a variation on the above issues. As mentioned above, hospital social workers—like their peers in the "service" sections of welfare departments—are *not* eligibility workers. Again, they have only a general and superficial knowledge of benefits rules and procedures, although this knowledge may be far more than the layperson's. Some hospitals, particularly those treating many indigents, arrange to have "Medicaid-only" eligibility workers placed in their facilities by the welfare office. Obviously, these persons will know far more about *Medicaid* eligibility than social workers or laypeople (for example, they can compute "spend downs"), but they will have no specialized knowledge of *other* programs (such as GA, AFDC, or Food Stamps), nor will they even know many details about *alternate* paths to Medicaid coverage (such as SSI).

Some hospitals also have their own employees such as "Hill-Burton coordinators" and "financial counselors"; similar to the welfare office's own eligibility workers, they are usually high-school-level clerks, to be relied upon only for routine cases in their rote specialties ("Medicaid-only", Hill-Burton, state-local "indigent care", or charity bill write-offs). Of course, as with the welfare office's eligibility and social workers, there will be an occasional exception to the rule here too; you may find someone who *has* successfully analyzed the local system *can* provide articulate and expert advice.

These real problems in negotiating the information gaps in local eligibility systems are, unfortunately, endemic; but then that's why this book was written.

The SSI and Medicaid Complexity

Since the most basic needs of PWAs are for income and access to health care, it follows that the central programs for their needs are SSI and Medicaid. And this is unfortunate, not only because both programs' eligibility rules are themselves incredibly complex, but because the interrelationships of SSI and Medicaid under the varying state procedures have produced a monstrous ganglion of rules, permutations, and exceptions. In fact, SSI and Medicaid are now viewed—at least privately—by their own policy staffs as nearly unadministerable. Up until 1972, everything was relatively simple: everyone on AFDC and the old state welfare programs for the aged, blind, and disabled got automatic Medicaid cards. About half of the states also covered the "medically needy": AFDC-type families and aged, blind, and disabled people who started out "too rich" for welfare, but whose medical bills "spent them down" to the Medicaid level.[1] But in 1972, Congress enacted Public Law 92–603, which created the SSI program and introduced a set of complex state options (some with burdensome anti-recipient biases) to the system:

  1. As a result of the addition of Title XVI (SSI) to the Social Security Act, states were required to allow Medicaid eligibility for SSI recipients (with one exception in #3 below) *but not necessarily automatically.*

1. Check the chapter on "Improving the System in Your State" to see if your state has a medically needy "spend down."

2. Section 1634 of the amended act provided for state-SSA contracts for "automatic" Medicaid for SSI recipients, *but only at state option.*

3. Section 209(b) of P.L.92–603 allowed states to retain some or all of the stricter Medicaid eligibility rules from their pre-SSI welfare programs (those rules governing income levels, asset levels, income disregard amounts, budgeting methods for living situations, and medical definitions of blindness or disability). This "loophole" was added to save the poorer, less liberal states from sudden Medicaid budget increases which would result if they had to give Medicaid to all those newly eligible under the more liberal SSI rules. However, Congress provided a "sop" to recipients in states which take this option: if the state did not already have a "spend down" rule for those "too rich" for Medicaid, it had to allow one if it took this "209(b)" option.

4. Section 1616 of the amended act allowed states to give higher incomes to their needy aged, blind, and disabled, by having the SSA simultaneously pay out "State Supplementary Payments (SSPs)" as part of, and on top of, the SSI payment. Thus, state-financed SSPs could, in effect, "raise" the SSI (and, therefore, the Medicaid) level in those liberal states wishing to be more generous. Unfortunately, *this feature, too, was made optional* for the states.

The changes made by P.L. 92–603, and the wide range of state options exercised under its provisions, introduced even more Byzantine complexities into the welfare system. And just for good measure, Congress added a series of arcane—yet all highly significant—technical changes to SSI, AFDC, Medicare, and Medicaid between 1973 and 1989. The discussion which follows in some sections of this book presupposes some general knowledge of these state options: "medically needy," "Title XVI," "1634," "209(b)," "1616," "2176" waivers, "poverty level" eligibility standards, and special, limited, "QMB" Medicare/Medicaid coverage. Those readers not versed in their own state's status may wish to glance over the appendices and the final chart in the closing section of the text to determine what options individual states have taken.

How Welfare Programs Count Income and Assets

Another set of concepts needs to be explained before we move on to program-by-program analysis. This involves levels of income and assets used to determine eligibility. An applicant's income is typically compared to a standard income eligibility level (almost always on a *monthly* basis): The applicant's income must fall below the level for the applicant to be eligible. (For *income* programs, then, the amount of the income benefit payment from the program is determined by *how much* an applicant's income is below the eligibility level: if John has *no* income, he gets a benefit equal to the amount itself of the eligibility level; if he has, say, $50 in income, he gets a benefit equal to the amount of the eligibility level *less $50*.) All of this is straightforward enough, until we come to the concepts of "disregards" and resulting "countable income" used in almost all programs. What this means is that benefit programs all have their own varying formulas to "disregard" (ignore the existence of) some income before they then compare the remaining "countable income" to the program eligibility level. The most widely known disregards are those of SSI: $65 and half the rest of earned income, then $20 of remaining income, is "disregarded" before the resultant "countable income" is compared to the eligibility level.

Related to "disregards" and "countable income" are the concepts of "exempt," "disregarded," and "countable" assets. Of course, almost all programs deny eligibility to those with assets—that is, "countable" assets—over an assets eligibility level. Some assets are "exempt" (for example, SSI exempts a *lived-in* home and a car to go to the doctor, no matter how valuable); others are "countable" (SSI "counts" liquid assets, and those over $2,000 generally render an applicant ineligible). Several other points need to be made about assets:

1. As in the old saying, "a house is not a home," SSI and most other welfare programs only exempt the value of a house *while the applicant or recipient actually lives in it;* real estate which is not lived in, or no longer lived in, almost always renders a person ineligible.

2. Generally, the SSI program does not care if an applicant with previously disqualifying assets gives them away, sells them to family or friends for less than fair market value, or squanders them, *but Medicaid and all state welfare programs do care*—they deny eligibility to those who so "dispose" of excess assets.

3. Medicaid can place a lien on and/or seek recovery from the estates and assets—even homes—of deceased applicants over 65 who had received "long term care," such as that in nursing homes and mental institutions. However, liens and recoveries from the estates of Medicaid patients *under* 65 are generally not permitted, unless there has been fraud. (Moreover, the homes of deceased or no longer "residing-in" Medicaid recipients of any age which are inhabited by legally married spouses or minor or "disabled" adult children—and, in some

cases, even siblings—are exempt from nonfraud recoveries or being counted as "excess" assets.)

Those who have been intrigued (or outraged) by the system complexities touched on by this introduction are invited to study carefully the final section of this book, "Improving the System in Your State."

Social Security Disability Insurance (SSDI)

Social Security Disability Insurance (SSDI) is an insurance program for disabled individuals who have worked and paid into Social Security. It pays variable monthly benefit amounts, depending on the applicant's work history, after a 5-month waiting period. Anyone applying for SSDI will also be helped to apply for SSI. SSDI uses the same disability rules as SSI.

1. Eligibility
- A covered worker must have a physical or mental impairment which has lasted, or is expected to last, *at least 1 year,* or which is expected to be fatal (see appendix D).
- The impairment must prevent the worker from engaging in *any substantial gainful activity* (SGA)—this means work earnings—which exists in the national economy of the United States.
- To be covered, a worker must have had earnings from which Social Security deductions were taken in at least 20 quarters (3-month periods) during the last 10 years—but there are shorter work period rules for very young workers.
- Those becoming disabled before age 22 can qualify from *parental* work records if a parent is dead, disabled, or retired.
- Certain widows, widowers, and divorced spouses are eligible for disability benefits on their deceased or former spouses' earnings records.
- AIDS, when documented by medical records showing "qualifying" conditions and opportunistic infections, is a disability according to SSDI guidelines (see appendix D–1a).
- AIDS-Related Complex (ARC) is not automatically considered a disability—but ARC patients with HIV-positive blood tests may qualify if ARC-related maladies such as long-term flu-like symptoms, fevers or night sweats, fatigue, wasting, malaise, severe diarrhea, depression, anxiety, confusion, memory impairment, paranoia, or substance abuse are cited on disability forms and questionnaires by applicants and their doctors as resulting in an inability to work. Psychological factors and a history of substance abuse (even if the applicant is currently in recov-

ery), when written up by applicants, mental health therapists, or substance abuse recovery counselors or sponsors, can be crucial in getting approval for ARC and other doubtful cases. Statements by applicants, therapists, friends, and co-workers about stress resulting from real or feared workplace discrimination are helpful too. ARC-only applicants who do not already have mental health therapists should seriously consider consulting (and, if necessary, paying) a therapist to secure a written evaluation to accompany their application packages (see appendices D–2, D–3, and D–4).

2. Benefits

· Benefits begin with the sixth full month of disability after "onset." Onset is considered to be the date that medical findings indicate the HIV-based pneumonic or disseminated opportunistic infection or disease resulted in an inability to work; an earlier onset date than that on which the applicant first sought medical care or was diagnosed may be established if it can be medically documented (see appendix D–1b).
· Monthly disability check is based on the worker's lifetime average earnings covered by Social Security (the average benefit in 1989 was about $550 a month).
· There are limits on earnings while receiving SSDI (generally $300 a month after certain deductions).
· SSDI recipients are eligible for Medicare after a 2-year waiting period.
· SSDI recipients *may,* depending on income eligibility rules of the state, be eligible for social services such as counseling, "meals-on-wheels," home chore aid, and transportation, through the "adult services" section of the welfare office. States provide these services for modest-income SSDI recipients, even if their incomes are somewhat too high for the SSI and Medicaid programs.
· SSDI recipients and pending applicants may (if needy) also be eligible for Emergency Assistance services such as the paying of delinquent rent, utilities, or mortgages (see Emergency Assistance section).

3. How and Where to Apply

· Apply at local Social Security office.
· Bring items shown in appendix E.
· People can apply by phone but only if someone later goes to the office to complete the paperwork.
· Applicants can apply for SSI and Medicaid (in *most* states; see Medicaid section) while at the Social Security office.

· Another person may assist or apply for incapacitated persons; this includes relatives, friends, social workers, and any other advocates.
· Apply *at once*—do not delay applying to gather documents and verifications; it could mean a loss of benefits. Supporting documents can be assembled later, if necessary.

4. Appeal Rights

· Denials, payment amount determinations, suspensions, reductions, terminations, or attempts to recoup "incorrectly paid" benefits can be appealed to a reconsideration, a hearing, an Appeals Council review, and, finally, to federal court, within 60 days after an adverse action. Appeals made *within 10 days* of each adverse action will temporarily prevent stoppage or reduction of benefits in most cases.
· Where SSA proposes to recoup alleged "overpayments" or "incorrectly paid" benefits, recipients can also request a "waiver" within 30 days of the SSA notice; this will also delay any recoupment from ongoing benefits until a determination is reached. SSA will waive recoupment if the recipient can show that he or she was not "at fault" (that is, didn't know the rules or all the facts due to such factors as ignorance, confusion, the complexity of the program, or illness) *and* that the recoupment would "defeat the purpose of the program" (which is to give disabled people money to live on; recoupment leaves them less to live on) or is "against equity and good conscience" (that is, is unduly harsh or unfair or financially hurts a recipient who relied on the correctness of the "overpayment") or that the overpayment is too small to be worth recouping. Even if a recipient fails to convince SSA to waive recoupment, he or she can still negotiate to have the "overpayment" deducted through small "installments"; SSI recipients cannot be made to pay more than 10% of income in recoupments. Finally, any SSA denial of a waiver or acceptable recoupment-deduction plan is *itself* appealable (see above paragraph).
· For reconsiderations and appeals, only attorneys or other advocates who are experienced in Social Security cases should be consulted. Free or inexpensive help from lawyers and other advocates is available from area neighborhood legal services, Legal Aid Societies, and many bar associations. SSA, the local welfare office, and senior citizens' agencies will also know of available resources.

5. Additional Information and Special Problems

· A person who is found to be medically disabled enough for benefits can lose them if he engages in "substantial gainful activity" (SGA)—work earnings of $300 or more monthly count as "SGA" and render an otherwise disabled person *ineligible*.

- The SGA rule can be waived (for those already receiving benefits for more than a year) for a 9-month "trial work period" and then a 15-month "extended period of eligibility" (after the first 3 of these 15 months SSDI checks will stop, but any Medicare coverage will continue).[1] Those returning to work should be sure to ask about "trial work period" and "extended period of eligibility" waivers of the SGA rule to keep their Social Security benefits.
- Applicants and their physicians must be very careful to allege the earliest possible *date of onset* of the disability. This date will be used to determine both the *future Medicare* eligibility date (that is, the 5-month and then the 24-month waiting periods will begin with this date) and the *retroactive Medicaid* eligibility date (for up to 3 months before the month of application). Applicants and their physicians often unthinkingly respond with the current date or first treatment date—but they should use the *earliest estimated* onset date.
- Continued salary paid to a no-longer-fully-productive employee is called "subsidized employment" by Social Security, and does not count as "SGA." Thus, where an employee continues on the payroll as a form of "disguised charity" by a compassionate employer, the date "SGA" ceases—and thus the start of the 5-month waiting period—can be set back to a date before paychecks actually stop. This will result in earlier SSDI payments.
- Smaller additional SSDI payments are made to disabled workers' minor children and to the other parent caring for them.
- The Social Security Administration's criteria for evaluation of AIDS appears in appendix D.
- SSDI—unlike other programs discussed in this handbook—is *not* a welfare-type program. It is paid to all covered, qualified persons, rich or poor.
- SSA can arrange to make SSDI payments to a "representative payee" for incompetent recipients; as a practical matter, interested advocates—rather than SSA—will have to locate volunteers to do this.

1. Normally, this "extended" Medicare for those continuing SGA after trial work periods lasts only up to 3 years. However, the 1990 Omnibus Budget Reconciliation Act will allow those reaching the 3-year limit to *purchase* Part A Medicare (but not Part B); moreover, since Part A premiums are very high ($234 monthly in 1988!), this law *requires* state Medicaid programs to pay the premium for those with incomes below 200% of poverty (about $1045 monthly in 1990).

· SSDI is not payable to otherwise eligible persons in prisons, but SSDI benefits for dependents are payable.
· SSDI benefits are raised each January 1 by the annual cost-of-living percentage.

Supplemental Security Income (SSI)

Supplemental Security Income (SSI) is a welfare program for poor people who are disabled, over 65, or blind. Eligibility determinations are made by the Social Security Administration. Anyone applying for SSI will also be helped to apply for SSDI and Medicaid. SSI uses the same disability rules as SSDI.

1. Eligibility

- A disabled person of any age must have a physical or mental impairment, preventing him or her from substantial gainful work, which is expected to last at least 12 months or to result in death (see appendix D).
- Applicant must be a U.S. resident or permanent resident alien.
- A car worth $4,500 or less is disregarded.
- $2,000 countable assets per individual are exempt. Countable assets or resources refers to savings, investments, worth of household belongings over $2,000 and, in some instances, burial plots and the *cash* (not face) value of life insurance policies.
- A car of any value is disregarded if it is used to go to a doctor.
- A *lived-in* home of any value is disregarded.
- In 1990, monthly "countable" income must be less than $386 per individual (countable income means all wages, pensions, interest, SSDI payments, *direct* money or in-kind gifts, but not loans or indirect medical, housing, or food assistance). See appendix B–1, however, for higher income levels allowed in states which "supplement."
- $65 and half of the rest of earned income is disregarded before comparing income to eligibility level.
- $20 of remaining income is also disregarded before comparing income to eligibility level.
- There is a lesser eligibility level (about $257 monthly in 1990) for those who live in other persons' homes and cannot prove that they pay their own proportionate share of rent and related expenses.
- AIDS, when documented by medical records showing "qualifying" conditions and opportunistic infections, is a disability according to SSI guidelines (see appendix D).

· As for SSDI, AIDS-Related Complex (ARC) is not automatically considered a disability—but ARC patients with HIV-positive blood tests may qualify if ARC-related maladies such as long-term flu-like symptoms, fevers or night sweats, fatigue, wasting, malaise, severe diarrhea, depression, anxiety, confusion, memory impairment, paranoia, or substance abuse are cited on disability forms and questionnaires by applicants and their doctors as resulting in an inability to work. Psychological factors and a history of substance abuse (even if the applicant is currently in recovery), when written up by applicants, mental health therapists, or substance abuse recovery counselors or sponsors, can be crucial in getting approval for ARC and other doubtful cases. Statements by applicants, therapists, friends, and co-workers about stress resulting from real or feared workplace discrimination are helpful too. ARC-only applicants who do not already have mental health therapists should seriously consider consulting (and, if necessary, paying) a therapist to secure a written evaluation to accompany the application packages (see appendices D–2, D–3, and D–4).

2. Benefits

· In 1990, SSI pays up to $386 for an individual, less "countable" income. Payment is one-third less for those who live in another's household. But see appendix B–1 for higher amounts paid in states which "supplement."
· SSI recipients get Medicaid too in just about all states—although in some states they must also visit the welfare office (see Medicaid section).
· SSI recipients are eligible for social services such as counseling, "meals-on-wheels," home chore aid, and transportation, through the "adult services" section of the local welfare office.
· SSI recipients or pending applicants may also be eligible for Emergency Assistance services such as the paying of delinquent rent, utilities or mortgages (see Emergency Assistance section).

3. How and Where to Apply

· Apply at local Social Security office.
· Bring items shown in appendix E.
· People can apply by phone but only if someone later goes to the office to complete the paperwork.
· Another person may assist or apply for incapacitated persons; this includes relatives, friends, social workers and any other advocates.

· Apply *at once*—do not delay applying to gather documents and verifications; it could mean a loss of benefits. Supporting documents can
be assembled later, if necessary.

4. Appeal Rights

· Denials, payment amount determinations, suspensions, reductions, terminations, or attempts to recoup "incorrectly paid" benefits can be
appealed to a reconsideration, a hearing, an Appeals Council review,
and, finally, to federal court, within 60 days after an adverse action.
Appeals made *within 10 days* of each adverse action will temporarily
prevent stoppage or reduction of benefits in most cases.
· Where SSA proposes to recoup alleged "overpayments" or "incorrectly
paid" benefits, recipients can also request a "waiver" within 30 days of
the SSA notice; this will also delay any recoupment from ongoing
benefits until a determination is reached. SSA will waive recoupment if
the recipient can show that he or she was not "at fault" (that is, didn't
know the rules or all the facts due to such factors as ignorance,
confusion, the complexity of the program, or illness) *and* that the
recoupment would "defeat the purpose of the program" (which is to
give disabled people money to live on; recoupment leaves them less to
live on) or is "against equity and good conscience" (that is, is unduly
harsh or unfair or financially hurts a recipient who relied on the
correctness of the "overpayment") or that the overpayment is too small
to be worth recouping. Even if a recipient fails to convince SSA to
waive recoupment, he or she can still negotiate to have the "overpayment" deducted through small "installments"; SSI recipients cannot be
made to pay more than 10% of income in recoupments. Finally, any
SSA denial of a waiver or acceptable recoupment-deduction plan is
itself appealable (see above paragraph).
· For reconsiderations and appeals, only attorneys or other advocates who
are experienced in Social Security cases should be consulted. Free or
inexpensive help from lawyers and other advocates is available from
area neighborhood legal services, Legal Aid Societies, and many bar
associations. SSA, the local welfare office, and senior citizens' agencies will also know of available resources.

5. Additional Information and Special Problems

· Most states can quickly grant General Assistance welfare to those
whose SSI applications are pending. They will usually accept a doctor's
statement on a welfare medical exam form. However, they ask SSI

applicants to agree to "pay back" the welfare out of their SSI awards when the SSI does go through. Because of bureaucratic bungling, these "paybacks" to welfare (out of the SSI awards of those who succeed) in some cases are never actually deducted. Therefore, all SSI applicants should be *sure* to apply for welfare as well, even if welfare or Social Security workers discourage these applications (see General Assistance section).

· Those with full-blown AIDS diagnoses (confirmed by a doctor via a brief note or even by telephone, stating that the patient has AIDS, noting HIV blood test results and identifying at least one opportunistic infection from the list in Appendix D–1c) qualify for "presumptive" disability determinations by Social Security—which means that the person with AIDS who is poor enough can receive SSI payments for up to 3 months while a *final* medical determination is being made. ("Presumptive disability determination" decisions and payments can be made by local offices, often within a few days.)

· Local offices not used to many AIDS cases may delay or hesitate to process quickly "presumptive disability" determinations; in these cases, applicants and their advocates should politely but firmly insist on sufficient action by showing a copy of appendix D–1b.

· Social Security disability standards and "subsidized employment" rules apply to SSI too (see Social Security section).

· However, even when an SSI applicant is exempted from the SGA limit, due to the "subsidized employment" loophole, the SSI recipient's "countable" income must still be below the eligibility level (for example, $386 monthly, after work disregards) for payments to continue.

· But any *Medicaid* for a person who is *already* an SSI recipient can continue indefinitely under Section 1619 of the Social Security Act, which exempts those who are *already* SSI recipients (but not *initial* applicants) from the SGA, "trial work period," and "extended period of eligibility" limits used in the SSDI program. This section thus allows working SSI recipients with continuing medical costs to have continued Medicaid coverage as if they were still on SSI (which they may no longer actually be if their earnings raise them over the SSI income level).

· Anyone not "living in own home" (owning or renting a home in own name, or having lease, rent receipts, or household bills for paying own way in home of lover, roommate or friend) will have the one-third reduction applied to the SSI eligibility level and payment. Therefore, no "not-in-own-household" SSI application should *ever* be filed without careful thought and preparation, since the one-third reduction of the SSI eligibility level (to $257 in 1990) can result not only in a lesser SSI check, but in *ineligibility* for any SSI (and, therefore, Medicaid) if the applicant has other small income. Thus, a PWA with a private disability insurance or SSDI benefit of $300 would be ineligible for both SSI and Medicaid under the $257/one-third-reduction/ "living-in-the-household-of-another" standard (even though he would be eligible under the full $386 SSI standard, were he living independently). This problem can be avoided when applicants submit notes from "roommates" stating that they are, in fact, paying their proportionate share of household expenses or, if they currently have little or no income, that their share of household expenses *is being loaned to them by the roommates,* and will gradually be repaid when benefits commence.[1]

· Disabled children, and even infants, can receive SSI. If they are living with parents, parental income is "deemed" to be available to a disabled child (after deducting amounts for work expenses and living allowances for parents and any other minor children in the home), and then compared to SSI one-person income level.

· "Deeming" of income also applies to a disabled person who has a spouse with income.

· Where a spouse or minor children of an SSI recipient also need help with living expenses, they should apply to the local welfare office for Aid to Families with Dependent Children (see AFDC section).

· Where an applicant has excess liquid assets (over $2,000) or non-lived-in real estate, SSA will sometimes grant "conditional eligibility" for a temporary period while the applicant disposes of the excess assets; SSA must then be repaid with the proceeds. Excess assets or proceeds *not* paid to SSA in this situation must not be given away, sold for less than fair market value, or squandered. If they are, the local welfare office will find an applicant ineligible for Medicaid when he applies there for it (see Medicaid section).

· The SSI eligibility and payment level drops to $30 monthly for those in medical institutions throughout a full month or more; where this results

1. This problem does not arise in California and a few other states where the state has tailored the SSP to "make up for" the one-third reduction for "living-in-the-house-hold of another" cases. Thus, uniform SSI/SSP levels apply no matter what the applicant's living arrangement (except for children living at home, married people, or those in group facilities). If your state has an SSP, call the local SSA office to find out whether the SSP compensates for the one-third reduction.

in ineligibility for SSI, and the patient's Medicaid coverage arose from receipt of SSI, he will have to reacquire Medicaid by applying to the local welfare office.

· SSA can arrange to make SSI payments to a "representative payee" for incompetent recipients; as a practical matter, interested advocates—rather than SSA—will have to locate volunteers to be so designated.

· SSI benefits are raised each January 1 by the annual cost-of-living percentage.

State Supplementary Payments (ssps)

Financial assistance for the disabled who need more than SSI income to live on is provided by State Supplementary Payment (SSP) programs which, in effect, "raise" the SSI level ($386 in 1990) by adding state welfare funds. Eligibility for an SSP also confers Medicaid eligibility. Naturally—at least for those not living in group homes—only rich, industrialized, liberal states choose to make these payments. Some states have no SSP programs at all; where SSPs are paid, the amount varies not only from state to state, but also by region and according to type of living arrangement.

A State Supplementary Payment (SSP) is always called just that by SSA when it administers the SSP as an "add-on" to the basic federal SSI program. (However, almost all recipients and most social workers and local welfare staff will refer to the combined total SSI/SSP program as "SSI"—they do not even realize that the basic federal SSI amount has had added to it a state-funded SSP.) In cases where states *separately* administer SSPs through their welfare offices, they sometimes use other terms as well: *public aid, auxiliary grants, state "pensions," income maintenance, public assistance, welfare, home relief, county relief,* and often, *Aid to Permanently and Totally Disabled* (APTD). The last term was the name of the welfare program for the disabled operated by the states before the creation of SSI in 1974.

1. Eligibility

· In almost all states, SSP programs have the same disability standards, asset levels ($2,000, *lived-in* home, car to go to the doctor), and income disregards ($20 general, $65 and half the remainder of earned) as SSI.[1]

· SSP income eligibility levels—against which an applicant's "countable" income is compared—are *higher* than the basic federal SSI level ($386 in 1990).

· SSP income eligibility levels—where a state chooses to pay them at

---

1. Except in "209(b)" states listed in Medicaid section, where *some* states' rules may be less generous than those of SSI.

all—vary according to the applicant's living arrangement, marital status, and sometimes, according to whether the applicant resides in a high- or low-cost zone in the state. The "living independently" and "living in board and care home" SSP levels are shown in appendix B–1. See also note 1 in SSI section.

· A few states' SSPs cannot be expressed as a flat, identifiable monthly income level; in these states, an applicant's "countable" income is compared to an individualized welfare budget level set up by the welfare office for the applicant's personal living arrangements (see appendix B–1).

2. Benefits

· Recipients receive SSP checks, up to income levels shown in appendix B–1, less any "countable" income.
· SSP recipients get Medicaid as well in just about all states.
· SSP recipients receive social services such as counseling, "meals-on-wheels," home chore aid, and transportation from the "adult services" section of the local welfare office.
· SSP recipients may also be eligible for Emergency Assistance services such as the paying of delinquent rent, utilities or mortgages (see Emergency Assistance section).

3. How and Where to Apply

· Apply at local Social Security office, where SSA pays the SSP (see appendix B–1). In this case, the SSI application also functions as the SSP application.
· Apply at local welfare office, where the state pays the SSP (see appendix B–1).
· Bring items shown for SSI in appendix E.
· Another person may apply for incapacitated persons; this includes relatives, friends, social workers and any other advocates.
· Apply *at once*—do not delay applying to gather documents and verifications; it could mean a loss of benefits. Supporting documents can be assembled later, if necessary.

4. Appeal Rights

· For SSA-administered SSPs, SSI appeal provisions are applicable (see SSI section).
· For state-administered SSPs, General Assistance appeal provisions are applicable (see General Assistance section).

5. Additional Information and Special Problems

- Almost all states have SSPs above the "living independently" level for disabled people living in group housing (see Board and Care Homes section).
- States are not required to raise their SSP levels each year by the cost-of-living rate (which SSI is required by law to do). Hence, each January 1, states make a wide range of SSP decisions: some raise them by the full cost-of-living percentage; some raise them by only part of the cost-of-living raise; some retain them at former dollar levels; some give other dollar-amount increases; most do nothing. (Note that SSP levels set forth in appendix B–1 are adapted from 1989 data; state responses to the January 1, 1990, SSI cost-of-living raise may thus alter these projections. You can verify federally administered SSP levels for 1990 by calling the local SSA office. For 1990 figures on state-administered SSPs, call the local welfare office.)

Aid to Families with Dependent Children (AFDC)

Aid to Families with Dependent Children (AFDC) is a federal-state welfare program which pays public assistance to *certain kinds* of low-income families. This is the program most people mean when they think of "welfare."

1. Eligibility

- Under federal law, eligible families must have at least one child under 18, and be deprived of one parent's care due to his or her death, absence from the home, or incapacity to work for at least 30 days.
- States generally use a *far more liberal* definition of "incapacity" than SSDI and SSI use for "disability."
- About half the states also now cover families whose highest-earning parent has been unemployed for more than 30 days; by October 1, 1990, all states will do so.
- Liquid assets cannot exceed $1,500; a *lived-in* home and a modest automobile are almost always allowed; cash value of life insurance and burial policies often counts against liquid asset levels.
- AFDC recipients must cooperate in legal actions for child support against absent parents.
- All AFDC recipients over age 16 must meet the state's work requirements unless they are either enrolled in approved schooling, found "incapacitated" by the state, or caring for a child under age 3 (age 6 in some states).
- A pregnant woman with no other child is eligible for a check in most states (if her pregnancy is verified on welfare medical exam form).
- A single child can also be eligible for a one-person check. For example, a child who was born in, but was removed from (or abandoned by) an AFDC-recipient family is placed in AFDC foster care (AFDC-FC) and given Medicaid, usually by the "child and family services" section of the welfare office. Similarly, a child removed from (or abandoned by) a non-AFDC parent is placed in non-AFDC foster care (non-AFDC-FC) and given Medicaid, also by the "child and family services" welfare workers. Welfare checks may or may not actually be payable, depend-

ing on the child's living arrangements. Children in hospitals for long stays—or their caretakers—may not get welfare checks, while children's welfare grants are paid as child-care compensation—sometimes inflated above the normal one-person AFDC level—to any foster parents with whom a child is placed. This eligibility arrangement is usually what applies in the cases of HIV-infected infants in inner city medical institutions (often known as "boarder babies") *even though more flexible, advantageous arrangements could be made for such children if they were placed on SSI—for which they often qualify medically* (see SSI and Board and Care Homes sections).

· Income eligibility and payment levels vary by family size, by state and even by region within states; income levels are almost always significantly lower than those for SSI.

· Some work-related expenses ($75 per month) and babysitting charges ($40 per week per child) are disregarded before income is compared to eligibility level. Some child support income is disregarded too.

2. Benefits

· Recipients get welfare checks based on "countable income" and family size.

· Even more generous disregards of earned and child-support income exist for those *already* on AFDC.

· All AFDC recipients get automatic Medicaid and child and family social services (counseling, "meals-on-wheels," home chore aid, transportation, homemakers, child care, job training) from the local welfare office; in almost all states AFDC applicants will be processed simultaneously for Food Stamps.

· All AFDC families "working their way off welfare" are given at least a 1-year extension of Medicaid and free or inexpensive child day care; some additional months' Medicaid is granted for those with only modest earnings.

· Non-disabled adults in AFDC families are eligible for free basic education, as well as for job training, search, and placement, and child day care services.

3. How and Where to Apply

· Apply at the local welfare office.

· When applying, bring items shown in appendix E.

· Another person may assist or apply for incapacitated persons; this includes relatives, friends, social workers, and any other advocates.

· Apply *at once*—do not delay applying to gather documents and verifications; it could mean loss of benefits. Supporting documents can be assembled later, if necessary.

4. Appeal Rights

· Every state has a system for a supervisory conference, a fair hearing, a review by the state director, and, finally, state or federal court action. Objections made within 10 days of each adverse decision will usually temporarily block termination or reduction of benefits; otherwise, the time limit is 30 days for appealing each adverse decision.

5. Additional Information and Special Problems

· Income eligibility budgeting is far less simple and straightforward than that of SSI; state complexities, variations, zonings, loopholes, and overrides often make it impossible to express an eligibility level as a set dollar amount. (Typical 1990 AFDC income eligibility levels in Mid-Atlantic states are in the range of $250 for a one-person family, $325 for two, $400 for three, $475 for four, and so on.)
· *Fathers,* as well as mothers, can qualify to head an AFDC family where the mother is the dead or absent parent.
· Where *either* mother *or* father is "incapacitated," the whole family can qualify.
· Where *either* mother *or* father has been the higher earner and becomes unemployed, whole family can qualify under the "unemployed parent" provision.
· SSDI, SSI, and Medicaid determinations of "disability" are automatically accepted for purposes of AFDC's "incapacitated parent" feature.
· States' "incapacity" medical standards are far more liberal than SSDI/SSI definition of "disability"; any doctor's statement on a welfare medical exam form is almost always accepted.
· To qualify for continued Medicaid and child care due to increase in earnings, AFDC recipients must show pay stubs and other documentation to a welfare worker—the extensions do not happen automatically.
· Where a parent receives SSI, the other parent and/or minor children can be eligible for AFDC.
· Where a child does not live with his or her parent(s), almost *any other relative* can qualify as "caretaker" and, if needy, receive both AFDC and Medicaid.

General Assistance (GA)

General Assistance is a welfare program operated by most—but not all—states and localities. It also goes by such other names as *general relief, home relief, public aid, public assistance, income maintenance, welfare, county relief,* and *municipal aid,* and it provides incomes to qualified poor persons who are not members of AFDC-type families or who are not (yet) disabled enough for SSI.

1. Eligibility
- States and localities have their own widely varying income and assets eligibility levels. Usually a *lived-in* home is allowed, but rules on income levels, automobiles and liquid assets are *much stricter* than those for SSI.
- Almost all states will require a written statement on the welfare medical exam form from a doctor about inability to work (for 30 days, 60 days, 90 days, or whatever time minimum the state requires), but the disability standards are *far more liberal* than for SSI.
- GA has few, if any, income disregards.

2. Benefits
- General Assistance payment amounts are *far lower* than those of SSI. (Typical 1990 GA income eligibility levels in Mid-Atlantic states are in the range of $200–$250 monthly.)
- Recipients *may* (depending on the state or locality) be eligible for social services (counseling, "meals-on-wheels," home chore aid, and transportation) from the "adult services" section of the local welfare office.
- General Assistance applicants can be processed simultaneously for Food Stamps in most states.
- General Assistance recipients in the large, rich, liberal, industrial states are usually given medical assistance on substantially the same basis as that on which SSI recipients are given Medicaid. Indeed, these "General Medical Assistance" programs are often indistinguishable from Medicaid itself, with even welfare workers referring to the program as "Medicaid," and with the same benefits package. Smaller or more rural

states often offer watered-down medical assistance (for example, access limited to public hospitals and clinics, or care only paid for as authorized on a funds-available, bill-by-bill basis) to their General Assistance recipients. And, of course, the *most* conservative states and localities simply have *no* General Medical Assistance at all (see Medicaid section and appendix C).

3. How and Where to Apply

- Apply at the local welfare office.
- Bring items shown in appendix E.
- Another person may assist or apply for incapacitated persons; this includes relatives, friends, social workers, and any other advocates.
- Apply *at once*—do not delay applying to gather documents and verifications; it could mean loss of benefits. Supporting documents can be assembled later, if necessary.

4. Appeal Rights

- Every state has a system for a supervisory conference, a fair hearing, a review by the state director, and, finally, state or federal court action. Objections made within 10 days of each adverse decision will usually temporarily block termination or reduction of benefits; otherwise, the time limit is 30 days for appealing each adverse decision.

5. Additional Information and Special Problems

- General Assistance can be paid to people who are needy and somehow incapacitated but not "disabled enough" for SSI. It is especially useful for those who "only" have ARC or who are awaiting SSI eligibility determinations, because state and local General Assistance programs have *more liberal* disability standards than those for SSDI and SSI.
- Anyone who has not yet begun receiving SSI benefits should be *sure* to apply for General Assistance too, *even* if SSI or welfare workers discourage such applications (see SSI section).
- Availability of General Assistance varies from state to state and even from county to county. Large, liberal, industrial states typically have statewide, or nearly statewide, comprehensive General Assistance programs. Southern and rural states, on the other hand, only have "state-authorized" General Assistance programs, funded at county option. As one might expect, only the more urban, liberal areas within rural states choose to run General Assistance programs—while there is simply no help at all in conservative rural areas.
- See appendix C for more details on state General Assistance programs.

Emergency Assistance (EA)

Emergency Assistance is a federally aided, state-run program to pay one-time extraordinary expenses for low-income families—even "intact" families—with children. Most states also give this help to low-income people found to be disabled for the purposes of SSDI, SSI, or Medicaid. The most liberal states even cover childless people who have not yet been declared disabled.

1. Eligibility
- Eligibility varies state by state, and even county by county.
- Many states limit eligibility to those receiving AFDC, SSI, or other welfare payments. A few states cover other persons facing financial emergencies, although it may be necessary to show how a medical disability caused the crisis.
- Most states have income and asset eligibility levels similar to those of SSI.
- Generally, Emergency Assistance can only be applied for once a year.
- Usually, some detailed review of the applicant's past money management as well as *future* budgeting plans will be involved.

2. Benefits
- Some states only pay for *certain types* of help.
- Emergency Assistance *can* (depending on the state and locality) include payments for:
  - utility arrears
  - utility reconnection/deposit charges
  - overdue rent/mortgage
  - overdue property tax
  - moving expenses
  - furniture storage
  - replacement or repair of damaged/stolen furniture and appliances
  - shelter and even hotel bills while homeless
  - meals while homeless
  - food vouchers

· replacement of stolen/lost SSDI, SSI or welfare checks
· first month's rent for new apartment
· rental deposits

3. How and Where to Apply

· Apply for Emergency Assistance at the welfare office; in larger cities there are usually 24-hour hotlines, intake offices, or shelters to handle night and weekend emergencies.
· Bring items shown in appendix E.
· Apply *at once*—do not delay applying to gather documents and verifications; it could mean loss of benefits. Supporting documents can be assembled later, if necessary.

4. Appeal Rights

· Every state has a system for a supervisory conference, a fair hearing, a review by the state director, and, finally, state or federal court action. Objections made within 10 days of each adverse decision will usually temporarily block termination or reduction of benefits; otherwise, the time limit is 30 days for appealing each adverse decision.

5. Additional Information and Special Problems

· Many Emergency Assistance programs will refuse help if an applicant's future expenses exceed his or her projected income (that is, they will not pay rent arrears for someone whose income is less than the amount of his or her rent). Those waiting for their SSDI, SSI, or ongoing welfare benefits to begin may be able to avoid this roadblock by securing written statements from Social Security or the welfare worker attesting to the estimated starting date and amount of these benefits, if this amount will be enough to meet future expenses. Similarly, some localities may accept written statements from parents, friends, or gay- or AIDS-related organizations that they will make payments "on behalf of" (*not* "to") the applicant, in order to make up for his or her future budget deficit. If John's ongoing SSI is to be $386, and he is now applying to EA to pay arrears on his $400 rent, EA won't pay arrears because his rent is greater than his income-to-be, unless, for example, his parents commit themselves to pay *at least* $14 monthly (the "deficit") to the landlord for him.
· See section on the Low Income Home Energy Assistance program for additional information about help with utility arrears.
· Most Emergency Assistance programs will deny help to those whose

incomes appear sufficient to have met ongoing basic needs, but who nevertheless find themselves in crisis through what the welfare office deems to be "mismanagement."

· Where there is no adequate Emergency Assistance program—or when an applicant has been found ineligible—the Red Cross, private charities, church groups, and even utility companies themselves will sometimes have limited assistance programs.

· While most localities providing shelter give low-cost hotel rooms or comparable semi-private accommodations to homeless *families with children,* they only have open-bay floor space in disused schools, armories, or warehouses for homeless single adults. However, PWAs with SSDI, SSI, or VA disability papers—or with notes from doctors, clinics, social workers, or others—may be able to convince Emergency Assistance or shelter workers to "upgrade" them to hotel rooms or the like on the grounds of medical necessity.

· New legislation and appropriations for shelter and related emergency care for the homeless—especially the *disabled* homeless—means that new programs are now becoming operative for the first time in many localities which previously had limited help or none at all.

· In all states, the Emergency Assistance program, or some similar health or welfare department program, will pay for burial of deceased persons for whom no one steps forward to assume responsibility.

· See appendix C for more details on state Emergency Assistance programs.

Food Stamps (FS)

The Food Stamps program is a federally funded and state-operated welfare program which helps poor people to buy food. Disabled individuals on SSDI or SSI are treated more generously than are others in the computation of eligibility. However, anyone not receiving those disability benefits could still be eligible for Food Stamps simply by being poor enough.

1. Eligibility

· No more than $2,000 in assets such as cash, savings, or stock. An automobile worth $4,500 or less or used by a disabled person, *lived-in* homes, personal belongings, and life insurance do not count as assets.

· In 1990, no more than $648 *gross* monthly income and $499 *net* monthly income.

· People receiving SSI or SSDI benefits or those over 60 need qualify only for the net income limits.

· Disabled individuals on SSDI or SSI and those over 60 are eligible for extra deductions for medical expenses and shelter costs when figuring net income.

· 20% of gross earned income is disregarded.

· $112 (for one person) of remaining income is disregarded. (See Food Stamp Computation Methodology.)

· *All* income—even income from welfare or SSI—is considered "gross income" in computing Food Stamp benefits.

· If able, applicants must meet certain work requirements.

2. Benefits

· Those found eligible are mailed monthly Food Stamp authorization forms, which they must present in person, together with their welfare office I.D. cards, for actual Food Stamp issuance at "redemption centers." These include welfare offices, banks, and, especially in large cities, storefront check-cashing facilities.

· In 1990, about $99 worth of Food Stamps (see Food Stamp Computation Methodology for amounts allowed outside the 48 states and D.C.) per month for those with no income; less for welfare, SSDI or SSI recipients, depending on income, shelter and medical costs (the greater the percentage of income taken up by shelter and medical costs, the greater the Food Stamp allocation). See appendix B–2 for *maximum* possible Food Stamp allotments for single SSI/SSP recipients, state by state, as estimated in early 1989.

· Persons receiving maximum payable *combined* SSI and SSP benefits in California and Wisconsin are not eligible for Food Stamps because the cash value of the stamps has been included in the SSI/SSP levels there.

· Food Stamps can be spent at most food stores, but only on food and plants or seeds to grow food; tobacco, alcohol, paper and cleaning products, pet food, and some ready-to-eat food cannot be purchased with Food Stamps.

Food Stamp Computation Methodology

(for separate one-person disabled household)

Start with gross total monthly income before deductions.
  Subtract 20% of any earned income. Result is countable earned income.
Subtract $112 of remaining income.[1]
Subtract *actually paid* medical costs (including Medicare and health insurance premiums) to the extent they exceed $35 monthly.
Result is net countable income.
Subtract 50% of net countable income from actual shelter cost (rent, proportionate share of rent or mortgage, plus taxes and utilities).
Subtract balance (if any) from net countable income.
Multiply result by 0.3, then round *up* to higher whole number.
Subtract result from $99.[2]
Result is Food Stamp allocation (but if the result is between $1 and $9, it is "rounded up" to $10).

Source: Author's conversation with Ann Gariazo, food program specialist, Food and Nutrition Service, U.S. Department of Agriculture, August 18, 1989.

1. Alaska, $191; Hawaii, $158; Guam, $224; Virgin Islands, $98.
2. Alaska, $123; Hawaii, $151; Guam, $146; Virgin Islands, $127.

· The amount of stamps received varies according to net income and the number of members in the food-sharing household.
· Food Stamp recipients are also eligible for some types of free food, such as cheese, under the TEFA program; however, they must ask for it expressly.

3. How and Where to Apply

· Apply at the local welfare office.
· When applying, bring items shown in appendix E.
· Apply *at once*—do not delay applying to gather documents and verifications; it could mean loss of benefits. Supporting documents can be assembled later, if necessary.
· Another person can assist or apply for incapacitated persons; this includes relatives, friends, social workers, and other advocates. Moreover, because of the need to physically present the monthly authorization form at redemption centers for actual Food Stamp issuance, PWAs may wish to specify someone they wish to authorize to do this for them—for example, roommates or "buddies"—as the program allows such designees to pick up disabled persons' stamps for them.
· Individuals applying for welfare are simultaneously processed for Food Stamps in most states.

4. Appeal Rights

· Every state has a system for a supervisory conference, a fair hearing, a review by the state director, and, finally, state or federal court action. Objections made within 10 days of each adverse decision will usually temporarily block termination or reduction of benefits; otherwise, the time limit is 90 days for appealing each adverse decision.

5. Additional Information and Special Problems

· If an applicant qualifies, Food Stamps will be available within 30 days (within 5 working days for qualified "emergencies").
· Anyone who shares a house or apartment with other people who are not relatives should apply as an individual, stating that the applicant does not purchase food and prepare meals with the roommate(s). If, however, the roommates share food purchases and preparation, and if the group applies as a household, then all members' assets and income will be considered together in determining eligibility. This, of course, could render an applicant ineligible if the other household members' incomes are even modestly above subsistence levels.

- Where certain relatives live together, all their income and assets will be added together (which could result in the applicant's ineligibility) *even if* they claim to buy and prepare food separately. This includes not only stereotypical "nuclear family" households, but also those households composed of adult siblings (and their spouses, if any) or even those in which an adult child has returned to live again in his or her parents' home. There is one loophole, however: where the *sibling* or at least *one* of the parents with whom the applicant lives is disabled or over age 60, the program will permit the applicant to submit notes from all concerned that they are separate food-households—and thus the applicant whose own income is sufficiently low can thereby be eligible for Food Stamps.
- Persons receiving meals through programs such as "meals-on-wheels" or from shelters and soup kitchens can have their Food Stamp allocations *reduced* (if they only receive *some* meals free) or *terminated* (if they receive *all* meals free) if they report such benefits to a Food Stamp worker.
- Because Food Stamp eligibility is recomputed fairly infrequently (usually every 6 months, once a year, or even less often), applicants certified on the basis of low General Assistance income levels (such as that before receipt of SSI) often continue getting that Food Stamp allowance *even after income rises with the start of higher SSI benefits.* Similarly, those given Food Stamp allowances based on SSI income often continue getting that SSI-based Food Stamp allowance even after income rises with the start of higher SSDI benefits (after the 5-month SSDI waiting period). Recipients who enjoy these unintended bonuses are, of course, expected to report such circumstances to their workers so that their benefits may properly be reduced; however, penalties for failing to do so are generally light—they usually amount to a future recoupment or reduction of Food Stamp allowances, at worst. Such actions, as is true of any welfare office actions, can be appealed (see SSI section for relevant arguments in any such appeal).
- Because there are no Food Stamp denominations in amounts less than $1.00, groceries return coins to recipients in making change for purchases less than $1.00. (Indeed, if the grocery store cash drawer does not contain Food Stamps in the right denominations, change is often given for amounts *more than* $1.00 in *bills*—even though this is technically prohibited.) Change-making allows recipients running low on money to convert unused Food Stamp coupons to cash: a recipient needing taxi fare to go to the doctor could make a series of candy bar

purchases with Food Stamps to secure sufficient cash for carfare. Moreover, in most inner-city areas one can easily arrange to convert Food Stamps to cash (at a discount), although this is illegal.

· See appendix B–2 for maximum possible monthly Food Stamp allowances for SSI/SSP recipients, state by state. These tables are based on living arrangements where the SSI/SSP recipient is paying substantial rent; with lesser rents, the Food Stamp allotment would also decrease.

Temporary Emergency Food Assistance (TEFA)

This federal program is designed to distribute surplus food to poor people. It is operated by local governments and nonprofit agencies.

1. Eligibility
· Anyone on welfare, SSI, Medicaid, or Food Stamps is eligible.

2. Benefits
· Free food packages including cheese, butter, dry milk, corn meal, flour, honey, and assorted other items.

3. How and Where to Apply
· Food is distributed through local agencies such as food banks, soup kitchens, churches, and other nonprofit organizations. There are often long lines and lengthy waits.
· Distribution and eligibility information is usually available at the welfare office.
· Bring proof of welfare, SSI, Medicaid, or Food Stamp eligibility.

Department of Veterans Affairs (VA) Benefits

The Department of Veterans Affairs offers both income support and medical care to certain qualified veterans. Services are available through VA hospitals, clinics, Veterans Outreach Centers, and regional offices throughout the country. Generally, veterans must have served at least 180 days on active duty and have been given honorable or general discharges. Dishonorable, bad conduct, and undesirable discharges almost always prevent eligibility for VA programs. Whether or not a disability is "service-connected" (that is, arising during or as a result of time on active duty) is also a key factor in VA programs.

A. Medical Benefits

1. Eligibility

- First priority for routine, nonemergency medical treatment is given to:
  - veterans with service-connected disabilities
  - veterans discharged due to disability
  - veterans receiving or eligible for disability compensation
  - former prisoners of war
- Second priority are those veterans without service-connected disabilities who allege exposure to nuclear explosions or to Agent Orange (that is, who once served in Southeast Asia), who can receive medical treatment if no other cause of their condition can be convincingly shown.[1]
- Third priority are veterans without service-connected disabilities but with annual incomes under $17,240 (in 1990), who are referred to as "Category A."
- Last priority are higher-income veterans *without* service-connected disabilities who are entitled only to emergency room treatment, for a clear medical emergency, until they can be stabilized for transfer elsewhere.
- Higher-income veterans without service-connected disabilities *may— solely at VA discretion*—be admitted for inpatient hospitalization or outpatient treatment, but only if space is available. Within this last

1. Neither VA regulations nor any appeals cases have so far defined the exact nature of this loophole, however.

priority class, veterans with annual incomes below $22,987 ("Category
B" in 1990) are admitted or treated before those with higher incomes
("Category C").

2. Benefits
· Inpatient hospital care.
· Outpatient hospital treatment.
· Clinic services.
· Inpatient and outpatient substance abuse programs.
· Psychotherapy and counseling.
· Outpatient pharmacy drugs (including AZT).
· Skilled and intermediate nursing facility care.

3. How and Where to Apply
· Apply at any VA hospital or clinic.
· Bring items shown in appendix E.

B. Compensation for Service-Connected Disabilities

1. Eligibility
· Compensation can be paid for injuries or illnesses arising from or
  during active duty service—even if caused or contracted off-duty, off-
  base, or on leave, no matter how short a time the veteran was on active
  service.
· Injuries or illnesses arising within limited time after discharge are
  presumed to be service-connected.
· Injuries or illnesses which would otherwise be considered service-
  connected are not compensable if they are caused by "willful misconduct" such as criminal acts, *drug abuse*, alcoholism, "intentional"
  attempted suicide by the sane and *venereal disease due to "illicit"
  sexual activity*.
· Nevertheless, the VA has not yet been known to deny disability
  compensation to those discharged with HIV infection, ARC, or AIDS.
· Compensation payments are not taxable, but they *are* "countable" by
  SSI, Medicaid, and other welfare programs, and thus can reduce those
  benefits or end eligibility for them altogether.

2. Benefits
· From about $79 monthly (10% rated disability), through about $441
  monthly (50% rated disability), up to about $1,574 monthly (100%

rated disability) in 1990, depending on medical determination by the VA; compensation payments are not means-tested like welfare, so rich and poor get the same benefits.

· Veterans with current disability ratings below 100%—for HIV infection contracted or first identified during active service—can be paid at 100% if recipients are found to be "unemployable." To this end, a case can be made on application that fear or prejudice or rapid *expected* onset of full-blown AIDS from what is only currently at the ARC or even "HIV-positive" stage renders a veteran "unemployable" *now* and thus 100% disabled *now*.

· Veterans can get a lesser compensation payment level raised temporarily to 100% for time in a hospital, if it is more than 21 days.

· Additional compensation is paid for spouses and minor children of veterans with disabilities rated over 30%.

· Medical equipment, prosthetic devices, and other such items are provided free of charge.

· Death compensation payments are made to spouses and children of veterans who die of service-connected disability; the amounts are tied to the veteran's military rank.

3. How and Where to Apply

· Apply at any VA hospital, clinic, outreach center, or regional office, or by mail to VA headquarters in Washington, D.C.

· Submit items shown in appendix E.

· Send Form SF–180 to National Personnel Records Center, 9700 Page Boulevard, St. Louis, MO 63132, for copies of military records. VA facilities stock copies.

· Consult staff of Veterans Outreach Center, Disabled American Veterans, or Vietnam Veterans of America *before* filing application.

· Apply *at once*—do not delay applying to gather documents and verifications; no benefits are payable for times before application date, even if applicant is otherwise eligible.

C. "Pensions" for Permanently and Totally Disabled Veterans (Whether or Not Disability Is Service-Connected)

1. Eligibility

· Veteran must have served during "wartime," *but not necessarily in the war zone.* "Wartime" is World War I, World War II, Korean Conflict (1950–1955) and Vietnam (1964–1975).

- Disability need *not* arise from time of active service.
- Veteran must be "totally and permanently disabled" (that is, for the remainder of life). Detailed rules are tied to complexities of VA's disability "ratings" system used for disability *compensation* system; however, those meeting the SSDI/SSI definition of disability will generally be eligible.
- Those who have lesser disability "ratings" but are found "unemploy-able"—as under the *compensation* system—can sometimes qualify as "permanently and totally disabled."
- Pensions, unlike compensation, are welfare-type, needs-based payments; nonwelfare income from other sources is, therefore, "count-able" under the VA pension program. The VA has no income disregards.
- "Countable" income must be below monthly basic pension amount plus applicable "housebound" and/or "aid and attendance" increments (see below); any assets other than a *lived-in* home and one car render a veteran ineligible.
- The VA does not count benefits from SSI, GA, or AFDC as "income" because these, too, are welfare-type payments. However, those pro-grams and Medicaid *do count* VA pensions as "income." By contrast, SSDI and any private pension or earnings *are* "countable income" for VA pension purposes (because these are *not* welfare-type payments).
- The "housebound" increment to the basic pension level requires that a veteran be rated 100% disabled and be permanently or substantially confined to his home, a hospital, a nursing home, a board and care home, or a hospice.
- The "aid and attendance" increment requires that a veteran be a nursing home or hospice patient; a board and care home resident; bedridden at home; unable to dress, eat, or go to the bathroom without help; in need of help with a prosthetic appliance; *or* unable to protect himself from "environmental hazards" without help.
- A veteran's disability, "housebound" status, or need for "aid and attendance" should be certified in writing by a *VA* doctor. Written statements by *non*-VA doctors, however, will also be considered as additional documentation.
- Veterans with service-connected *compensation* payments which are less than *pension* levels (with or without "housebound" and/or "aid and attendance" increments)—and who have served in "wartime" and are now permanently and totally disabled—are also eligible to have the higher pension payments replace their compensation benefit.

2. Benefits

· Up to $563 monthly (in 1990), less any other "countable" income, for basic pension.

· Additional amounts for veteran's spouse or minor children, less "countable" income.

· Up to $126 *more* monthly (in 1990), less any other "countable" income, if veteran is also medically determined to be "housebound."

· Up to $213 *more* monthly (in 1990), less any other "countable" income, if also medically determined to be in need of "aid and attendance" care. This "aid and attendance" payment, unlike the basic pension, "housebound" increment, and dependent allowances, is *not* "countable" by SSI or Medicaid.

· Many—if not most—PWAs should be able to qualify for the "housebound" and "aid and attendance" payments; the VA does *not* require that "aid and attendance" payments *actually be spent* on such services. This is relevant especially for PWAs with volunteer "buddies" or who are in need of or receiving home health, chore, or homemaker services from volunteers, health insurance, Medicare, Medicaid, or "adult social services" programs.

· "Death pensions" are payable to a spouse or children of a deceased veteran pension recipient. These, too, are welfare-type, need-based payments, and nonwelfare income from other sources (such as Social Security, pensions, or earnings) is "countable."

3. How and Where to Apply

· Apply at any VA hospital, clinic, outreach center, or regional office, or by mail to VA headquarters in Washington, D.C.

· Submit items shown in appendix E.

· Consult staff of Veterans Outreach Center, Disabled American Veterans, or Vietnam Veterans of America *before* filing application.

· Apply *at once*—do not delay applying to gather documents and verifications; no benefits are payable for times before application date, even if a veteran is otherwise eligible.

D. Community Residential Home Care and Adult Day Services Programs

Although it does *not* make payments directly for them, the VA provides placement, quality-of-care monitoring, and ongoing medically oriented social services in community residential home care facilities (board and care home-type residences)[2] and adult day services programs (socially supportive "day care" on the model of day-long senior citizens' center programs) to senile, infirm, chronically ill, handicapped, or socially isolated veterans who have been accepted and are current patients in or at VA Medical Centers.

1. Eligibility

- The veteran (whether or not his illness is service-connected, whether or not he has served in "wartime," or whether or not he is eligible for compensation or pension) must be a current patient at a VA Medical Center.
- It is the VA Medical Center social services staff which must determine that a veteran is senile, infirm, chronically ill, handicapped, or socially isolated, and that he is in need of the program. The same staff must refer him to the program.
- The criterion for being a "current" VA Medical Center patient means, in practice, that mostly only "service-connected" veterans who are admitted to routine, ongoing care are generally considered for programs. *Theoretically,* however, *any* veteran (even one ordinarily without sufficient medical priority, such as service-connected status, but who nonetheless manages to be accepted as a VA patient) can receive these services.
- The veteran need not be eligible for compensation or pension (with or without "housebound" or "aid and attendance" supplements); however, his underlying medical or social condition must be *comparable* to the disability criteria of compensation and pension programs.

2. Benefits

- Placement in VA-operated or VA-sponsored or -approved community residential home care facilities and adult day services programs.
- Monitoring by the VA of the quality of care and accommodations.
- Continuing medically oriented VA social work services.
- Protected, supervised, and home-like care, meals, and assistance with daily living activities, as appropriate.
- VA-provided transportation, as needed, to planned activities and to medical care.
- Continuing treatment by the referring VA Medical Center (whatever the veteran's medical priority would otherwise be). These VA programs do

2. See board and care homes section.

not *themselves* pay a veteran's fees for community residential home care or adult day services; the veteran does that with his compensation, pension, SSDI, SSI, SSP for Board and Care, or other income. The VA *will* assist the veteran in applying for these benefits.

3. How and Where to Apply

- Apply to social worker or workers at the relevant VA Medical Center to which you have been admitted for medical care (see subsection A).
- Submit items shown in appendix E, if again asked to do so.
- Request VA assistance or referral in applying to non-VA income programs, if necessary.

E. Appeal Rights

- Any veteran, or veteran's survivor, who is denied eligibility or benefits may appeal within 1 year to the VA regional office; if the applicant is still dissatisfied, he or she may take an appeal within 60 days to the Board of Veteran Appeals, whose decision can *then* be further appealed within a year to the Court of Veterans' Appeals.
- Where VA proposes to recoup alleged "overpayments" or "incorrectly paid" benefits, recipients can also request a "waiver" within 30 days of the VA notice; this will also delay any recoupment from ongoing benefits until a determination can be reached. VA will waive recoupment if the recipient can show that he or she was not "at fault" (that is, did not know the rules or all the facts due to ignorance, confusion, complexity of the program, or illness), *and* that the recoupment would "defeat the purpose of the program" (which is to give disabled people money to live on; recoupment leaves them less to live on) or is "against equity and good conscience" (is unduly harsh or unfair or financially hurts a recipient who relied on the correctness of the "overpayment") or that the overpayment is too small to be worth recouping. Even where a recipient fails to convince the VA to waive recoupment, he or she can still negotiate to have the "overpayment" deducted through small "installments." Finally, any VA denial of a waiver or acceptable recoupment-deduction plan is *itself* appealable (see terms of above paragraph).
- Medical treatment eligibility and admission *policies* are not subject to appeal; only *factual determinations* under those policies are appealable.
- Federal law prohibits veterans from paying lawyers more than $10 to

handle their cases. However, normally paid legal representation *is* allowed for cases appealed to the Court of Veterans' Appeals, or referred by it for further adjudication.

· Free, expert advocacy is available from the following:
  · Veterans Outreach Centers (check the government section of the phone book, or call the 800 number for the VA and ask for the nearest center);
  · Vietnam Veterans of America (call directory assistance or (800) 852–2369 for the nearest branch);
  · and Disabled American Veterans (call directory assistance or (202) 554–3501 for the local branch).

F. Additional Information and Special Problems

· Any veteran discharged with HIV infection, ARC, or AIDS who is denied disability compensation on grounds that the illness was caused by "misconduct" (alleged drug abuse or "illicit" sexual activity) should contact Vietnam Veterans of America at (202) 797–8366 for advice and assistance.

· Veteran's disability compensation payments and pensions (except for the pension's "aid and attendance" increment) are considered "countable" income by SSI, welfare, and Medicaid—PWAs dependent on Medicaid for medical care need to consider carefully the possible loss of Medicaid which can result from receiving VA compensation and pensions (which are often *above* welfare, SSI, and Medicaid levels).

· Health insurance plans of non-service-connected veterans receiving VA medical care will be billed.

· Non-service-connected veterans with annual incomes of more than $22,987 (in 1990) will be billed for at least part of VA medical care (except for amounts covered by any health insurance they may have).

· VA Medical Centers can use their own funds to establish and operate community residential home care and adult day services programs, and some do so; often, however, patients are placed in programs run by state or local agencies, nonprofit groups, or even private operators. For a Medical Center to fund the *establishment* of a new or expanded community residential home care or adult day services program, a specific mandate would be required in the annual VA appropriations bill.

· *All* veterans, non-service-connected veterans and even some of those with "bad discharges," may receive counseling, individual and group therapy, and substance abuse information and referral services from the VA's Veterans Outreach Centers.

· The VA also arranges for free flags and honor guards for burial, national cemetery plots (if space is available) and, in some cases, small one-time payments to survivors of deceased veterans, whether or not the deceased were eligible for other VA benefits.

· Disabled VA patients and compensation or pension recipients may also be eligible for social services such as counseling, "meals-on-wheels," home chore aid, and transportation, from the "adult services" section of the local welfare office.

AZT and Other Drug Programs

AZT Program

A state-administered emergency fund to pay for the drug Retrovir (zidovudine), also known as AZT—as well as for alpha interferon and aerosolized pentamidine—for low-income AIDS patients was established by the U.S. Public Health Service for fiscal 1987, 1988, 1989, and 1990. Legislation is planned to continue funding for the program in subsequent years. Each state receives funds in proportion to its share of all U.S. AIDS cases and establishes its own income eligibility rules.

1. Eligibility
- Low-income persons who are not completely covered by Medicaid or private insurance or whose state Medicaid program does not cover these drug costs are eligible for assistance.
- At a minimum, drugs are free to those with income below or up to the poverty level (in 1990, about $522 monthly for one person), with partial assistance based on sliding scales as income rises. However, many states' income rules are far more generous. Asset levels vary.

2. Benefits
- The fund will cover the costs of AZT, alpha interferon, and aerosolized pentamidine. (Several states, however, only cover AZT.)

3. How and Where to Apply
- Information and application forms are generally available at county and city health or welfare departments for localities with large numbers of AIDS patients.
- Otherwise, each state has a statewide office and hotline where inquiries can be made and from which application forms can be ordered (see appendix A).
- Bring items shown in appendix E.
- Apply *at once*—do not delay applying to gather documents and ver-

ifications; it could mean loss of benefits. Supporting documents can be assembled later, if necessary.

State and Local Drug Programs

In addition to the AZT Drug Program, nine states and some localities have their own drug assistance programs—which often have income eligibility levels *more liberal* than those of Medicaid and cover most types of prescription drugs—not just AZT. The states with drug assistance programs for persons not on Medicaid are Connecticut, Delaware, Illinois, Maine, Maryland, New Jersey, New York, Pennsylvania, and Rhode Island. In these states, the AZT program hotlines should have information and application forms for these programs (see appendix A). If there are any *local* drug programs (which a number of more liberal local governments do fund), they will be known to local health or senior citizens' agencies; the local welfare office's "adult services" staff may also know about them.

Other Sources of Drug Assistance

DISCOUNT DRUG-BUYERS' CLUBS
Groups of PWAs and their advocates in several parts of the country have banded together to buy both experimental and as-yet-unapproved drugs, as well as some regular drugs, at discounts obtained through bulk purchasing. Further information about these programs is available from the People With AIDS Health Group in New York: (212) 532-0363.

AMERICAN ASSOCIATION OF RETIRED PERSONS (AARP)
MAIL-ORDER PHARMACY
The AARP operates a mail-order prescription drug service *with substantial discounts* both for its regular members (who must be over age 50) and for its "associate members" (who may be *under* age 50). Send name, address, birthdate, and $5.00 annual dues to:

American Association of Retired Persons (AARP)
Membership Processing Center
P.O. Box 199
Long Beach, CA 90801-9989

DISCOUNTS FOR THOSE WITH DRUG INSURANCE

Stadtlander's Pharmacy (address: 3600 Laketon Road, Pittsburgh, PA 15235) accepts health insurance which covers such AIDS drugs as AZT and others and *accepts the health insurance payment as payment in full. Thus, the patient is not billed for the coinsurance* (which could be 20%, 50%, or more)! Call (800) 238–7828, (800) 231–7828 in Pennsylvania, for information on ordering.

Eyre's Pharmacy (address: 1932 Martin Luther King, Jr. Avenue, S.E., Washington, DC 20020) *waives both the coinsurance and the deductible* for orders of AZT and some other AIDS drugs for those with health insurance covering drugs. Call (202) 678–2711 for ordering information.

FREE DRUG AND MEDICAL CARE RESEARCH PROTOCOLS

The federally run National Institutes of Health (NIH), the Department of Veterans Affairs (VA), other federal and state health agencies, and private research institutions provide free AIDS-related drugs, and sometimes medical care, to those participating in research studies and protocols—not only at their own facilities, but at other medical institutions throughout the country. In some cases, overall AIDS treatment, as well as the particular drug or procedure under study, is provided free of charge. Contact major medical institutions to find out about programs available in local areas, or call NIH at (800) 342–AIDS or (800) TRIALS–A.

Medicare

Medicare is a federal health insurance program for certain disabled and aged people.

1. Eligibility

- Anyone who has been entitled to Social Security Disability Insurance (SSDI) benefits for 2 years, or who is over 65, or who experiences permanent kidney failure.

2. Benefits

- Medicare Part A–Hospital Insurance pays for:
  - Inpatient hospital care for 60 days, if medically necessary, after 1990 annual deductible of $592; then, all but $148 per day for next 30 days; and finally, all but $296 per day for next 60 days of *lifetime reserve* (which can only be used once). Only 190 days of mental hospital care per lifetime.
  - Inpatient skilled nursing facility care, after hospital stays of at least 3 days (this does *not* mean *any* "nursing home"; it means only those offering *skilled, professional nursing* and related care for those who need it) for up to 100 days per year, with co-payments of $74.00 per day for days 21 through 100.
  - Home health care visits, by registered nurses or other medical professionals, but *not* simply housekeeping or personal care (except as an adjunct to professional medical services); in 1990, these visits may take place up to 4 days per week over a period of up to 3 weeks of care per illness, with no deductible or copayment for those leaving the hospital.
  - Hospice care for up to two 90-day periods and one 30-day period.
- Medicare Part B–Medical Insurance, after $75 annual deductible, pays 80% of *allowable* charges for:
  - Physician's services
  - Outpatient hospital services and therapies

- Other services (such as tests, transportation, and equipment) not covered by Part A
- 100% of allowable charges (except for $75 deductible) for *non-post-hospital* home health care, up to 4 days per week for up to 3 weeks of care
- 62.5% of psychiatrists', psychologists', and licensed clinical social workers' services (with no dollar or visit limit)
- Medicare Part A is free, but Part B is partially paid for by the individual; the monthly premium, $28.60[1] in 1990, is automatically deducted from Social Security checks.
- Medicare Parts A and B will *not* cover:
  - Charges billed at amounts above those in the Medicare *allowable* fee schedule
  - Services provided by organizations or individuals not Medicare-approved and participating
  - Intermediate nursing home care
  - Custodial care in any setting (nursing home or home health care which anyone can render, such as housekeeping, cooking, cleaning, grooming, or personal care)
  - Care that is not reasonable or necessary and services or supplies not generally accepted (such as acupuncture or experimental drugs or treatments)
- Hospice benefits have no deductibles and cover inpatient care, home health care, "significant other" counseling and support services, and almost all of the charges for drugs.

3. How and Where to Apply

- Those receiving Social Security Disability Insurance benefits will automatically be enrolled when the 2-year waiting period is over.
- Others should apply at the local Social Security office.

4. Appeal Rights

- Denial and terminations of *eligibility* can be appealed to a reconsideration, a hearing, an Appeals Council review, and, finally, to federal

---

1. Because Congress repealed the Medicare Catastrophic Coverage Act so late in 1989, SSA will probably be unable to correct its computers to prevent the formerly planned additional "catastrophic" premium deduction of $5.30 monthly from SSDI checks (for Medicare eligibles) before mid-1990. Refunds are to be made to those whose checks undergo this erroneous deduction.

court, within 60 days after an adverse action. Appeals made *within 10 days* of each adverse action will temporarily prevent stoppage or reduction of benefits in most cases.

· For reconsiderations and appeals, only attorneys or other advocates who are well experienced in Social Security cases should be consulted. Free or inexpensive help from lawyers and other advocates is available from area neighborhood legal services, Legal Aid Societies, and many bar associations. SSA, the local welfare office, and senior citizen agencies will also know of available resources.

· Medicare recipients receive notices of all claims payments and nonpayments; these decisions can also be appealed, and information about how to do so is printed on payment notices.

· Hospitalized Medicare patients dissatisfied with the quality of their care or with the hospital's discharge or placement arrangements should appeal *at once* to the Peer Review Organization serving their area (see appendix L). Pre-discharge complaints will delay and possibly (if upheld) cancel any poorly planned discharge and force the hospital to make adequate post-discharge housing arrangements for those who need them.

5. Additional Information and Special Problems

· In many instances, someone can be on both Medicare and Medicaid; in this case Medicaid will pay that part of medical bills not paid by Medicare as well as the patient's monthly Medicare premium. The beneficiary need do nothing to arrange this once he has been found eligible for Medicaid; Medicare and Medicaid arrange it automatically. It is called the "Buy-In." In such a case, the Part B premium, of course, ceases being deducted from the SSDI check.

· Medicare's "allowable charges" fee schedule for doctors and others is *far* below what is charged to and paid by private patients and health insurers. This means that if the doctor or other provider refuses to accept the Medicare "allowable charge" as payment in full (and many do), the patient will have to pay not only 20% of the "allowable charge," but *all* of the billed amount above that level.[2] Therefore, it is

2. When doctors "take assignment" (that is, bill Medicare directly themselves), federal law has long required them to accept the Medicare rate. But when they refuse "assignment," they have been able to bill the patient for more than the approved charge (except for a complex and relatively unenforceable limit imposed during the mid-1980s). However, the 1990 Omnibus Budget Reconciliation Act limits even "nonassignment" doctors in billing for balances over the Medicare rate (no more than 125% of the rate in 1991, 120% in 1992, and 115% in 1993 and thereafter). Of course, this law will not prevent doctors from simply refusing to treat Medicare patients at all.

vitally important that patients find out whether medical providers accept the Medicare fee schedule. Social Security offices and local senior citizens' agencies maintain lists of Medicare-participating doctors; those interested can also secure a list by calling (800) 234–5772.

· Hospitals which once received Hill-Burton grants (even if they no longer must dispense free care—see Hill-Burton section) are *required* to provide Medicare-participating staff physicians to their patients.

· Some states—including several New England states—have general medical licensure laws requiring *all* doctors—even those who do not wish to do so—to participate in Medicare and to accept the Medicare fee schedule as payment in full. Such laws are being proposed by health advocacy groups in many other states (see appendix G–2), usually over the opposition of the medical profession. (See also note 2.)

· Those whose opportunistic infections or other medical conditions lead to serious kidney malfunction or failure may be eligible for Medicare with only a 3-month waiting period (the 2-year waiting period does not apply in this case).

· Medicare—unlike other programs discussed in this handbook—is *not* a welfare-type program. It is offered to all covered, qualified persons, rich or poor.

· See Medicaid section for details on the "Qualified Medicare Buy-In" (QMB), through which *certain poor* Medicare beneficiaries can have their Medicare premiums, deductibles, and coinsurance paid by Medicaid *even* if they are otherwise ineligible for *full* Medicaid eligibility in their states.

· Where a Medicare patient has private health insurance as well (such as a privately purchased individual plan or an employer-based plan continued after the employment ceased), Medicare pays first, then the insurance pays second. Moreover, even if the private plan ordinarily pays more than Medicare (and most do), *its rate schedule will conform to Medicare fees for joint patients.* Hence, even those with health insurance, because their plans must adopt Medicare fees, sometimes experience problems in securing doctors willing to accept the fee scale.

· If, by some chance, a Medicare patient is covered by an employer-based plan *for active employees,* the private plan pays first and then Medicare is secondary.

· Medicare claims are not processed by the government; instead, private insurance companies do this under contract. Names and addresses of these contract claims processors—called "carriers"—are provided in appendix M.

Medicaid

Medicaid is a federal-state program[1] which can pay most types of medical expenses for *certain* kinds of persons who have incomes and assets below state-set poverty levels, or (in most states) whose incomes fall to those poverty levels through *incurred* (but not necessarily *paid*) medical expenses. The kinds of poor persons covered are those in AFDC-*type* families (see AFDC section), those who meet the SSI/SSDI medical definition of blindness or disability (see Appendix D), pregnant women, those under age 7 or over age 65, and some or all persons (depending on the state) between age 7 and age 21.

1. Eligibility

· Under federal law, states give Medicaid to those who receive Supplemental Security Income (SSI) and Aid to Families with Dependent Children (AFDC) welfare payments. The 1990 income level for SSI is $386 per month but it is higher in states which "supplement" (see appendix B–1). AFDC levels vary widely among states.

· Everyone who is receiving SSI will automatically be eligible in "1634" states, although in "Title XVI" and "209(b)" states SSI recipients will have to apply to welfare offices for Medicaid (see Introduction). AFDC recipients are automatically eligible everywhere.

· A few states give *all* Medicaid services to disabled people with "countable" incomes above SSI, SSP, or ordinary Medicaid levels but below the national poverty level ($522 per month in 1990). These states include Florida, New Jersey, Rhode Island, and the District of Columbia; several other states plan to do so. Beginning in 1990, *all* states must *at least* pay Medicare premiums, coinsurance, and deductibles for Medicare beneficiaries with "countable" income below about $470 monthly and liquid assets below $4,000 *even* if they are not eligible under the state's *regular* Medicaid rules for remaining Medicaid services. Of course, people who also meet the state's *regular* Medicaid eligibility rules would also get coverage of those Medicaid services not

1. The program is called "Medi-Cal" in California; it is called "AHCCCS" (pronounced "access") in Arizona.

56

NOT ELIGIBLE FOR MEDICAID
DUE TO "EXCESS INCOME"
OR BECAUSE YOU WORK?
(BECAUSE YOUR SOCIAL SECURITY OR OTHER PENSION IS OVER
THE LEVEL ALLOWED FOR SSI OR FOR PUBLIC ASSISTANCE?)

YOU CAN STILL
GET MEDICAID!!!

HERE'S HOW IT WORKS . . .

SAY THE MEDICAID ELIGIBILITY LEVEL IS $5,000 AND YOUR
INCOME IS $6,000. THIS MEANS THAT YOU HAVE
"EXCESS INCOME" BY $1,000.

BUT, ONCE YOU RUN UP MEDICAL BILLS OF $1,000 YOU
CAN SUBTRACT THE BILLS FROM YOUR INCOME, AND MAKE
IT LOW ENOUGH FOR MEDICAID! THIS WAY OF BECOMING
ELIGIBLE IS CALLED

"SPEND DOWN"

WHEN YOU USE "SPEND DOWN" TO GET MEDICAID,
COVERAGE CAN LAST MONTHS!!!

YOU DON'T HAVE TO PAY THE BILLS YOU USE IN
YOUR "SPEND DOWN" . . . YOU JUST HAVE TO
INCUR THEM!

ASK ABOUT "SPEND DOWN" NOW!!

SOURCE: Written and used by author in educating indigent hospital patients about Medicaid (1985).

covered *at all* by Medicare (for example, outpatient drugs or care in most nursing homes). This special feature is called the Qualified Medicare Buy-In ("QMB"), and the monthly income level for it will increase each year.

· Most states include other Medicaid-type people (such as those disabled according to SSI/SSDI definition) whose incomes are too high to begin with but whose *incurred* (but not necessarily *paid*) medical bills reduce their incomes to the state's ordinary Medicaid eligibility level. The deducting of incurred medical bills is called the "spend down" in almost all states; other states use terms like "cost share," "patient pay," "deductible," or "client participation" for this way of becoming eligible.[2] Anyone denied Medicaid due to "excess income" should ask the

2. Unfortunately, in "spend down" states, those with excess income must spend down to the *ordinary, general* Medicaid level, rather than to the usually higher, special "poverty/QMB" Medicaid level.

welfare worker about this method for becoming eligible. The "spend down" is *not* available at all in the following states: Alabama, Alaska, Colorado, Delaware, Georgia, Idaho, Mississippi, Nevada, New Mexico, South Carolina, South Dakota, Texas, and Wyoming.

· In Indiana, Ohio, and Missouri, the "spend down" is available to the aged, blind, and disabled, but not to other Medicaid applicants.

· In applying for Medicaid only, aged, blind, and disabled persons are accorded the income disregards of the SSI program,[3] while families and children receive the AFDC income disregards.

· Modest liquid assets (usually at least $2,000, as under SSI), an automobile and a *lived-in* home are allowed.[4]

· Medicaid uses the same disability standards as SSDI and SSI (see appendix D) and the same family definition, "incapacity," and "unemployed parent" rules as AFDC (see AFDC section).

2. Benefits

· Recipients are given plastic or paper Medicaid cards with which to purchase covered services from participating providers; cards are used similarly to major credit cards. However, *cash* outlays by patients are *never* reimbursed: Medicaid functions, in effect, as a "charge" plan.

· Medicaid covers the following services in almost all states:
  · Care in skilled and intermediate nursing homes
  · Inpatient hospital services
  · Outpatient hospital services
  · Clinic health services
  · Laboratory and X-ray services
  · Hospice services (in about half the states)
  · Home health services of registered nurses or other medical professionals, but *not* simply housekeeping or personal care
  · Physician services
  · M.D. psychiatrist services
  · *Some* states cover services of licensed psychologists and psychiatric social workers
  · Premiums, coinsurance, and deductibles for poor, disabled, and aged

3. Except in "209(b)" states (see Where SSI Recipients Apply for Medicaid, by State), where *some* states' rules may be less generous than those of SSI.

4. As is true of income disregards, some "209(b)" states may have less generous rules about assets than those of SSI.

people who are *also* on Medicare. This is called the "Buy-In."[5]

· Ambulance service
· Mass-transit tokens, taxi vouchers, and handicapped van service to get to medical care in some states
· Outpatient prescription drugs (including AZT, except in Alabama, Arkansas, Colorado, Texas, and Wyoming)
· "Personal home care attendants" (non-professional level), when ordered in writing by a doctor, in many states; however, there is an attendant shortage due to the low rates they are paid by Medicaid.
· "Home and community-based services," issued to the state by HHS under a "2176 waiver," to enable Medicaid to cover a wider range of services that is not regularly available in the state (such as enhanced home health care, personal care attendant, chore aid, homemaker, and other supportive services, often under broadened eligibility rules) for PWAs and other disabled and aged people. California, Florida, Hawaii, Illinois, New Jersey, New Mexico, North Carolina, Ohio, Missouri, and South Carolina already have such waivers; other states are considering seeking them. Legislation passed in 1988 also offers states the option of providing enhanced "home and community-based services" to PWAs under age 5, even without a waiver.
· Medicaid recipients are also eligible for social services such as counseling, "meals-on-wheels," home chore aid, and transportation, through the "adult services" section of the welfare office.

3. How and Where to Apply

· All states process applications at the local welfare office.
· In "1634" states, SSI eligibility automatically confers Medicaid eligibility. In "Title XVI" and "209(b)" states, SSI applicants or recipients apply for Medicaid at the welfare office (see Where SSI Recipients Apply for Medicaid, by State).
· Medicaid can be retroactive for up to 3 months before the month of application *if* expressly asked for and *if* the applicant met the SSDI/SSI

5. Medicaid *must* pay uncovered parts of the Medicare benefit package, but not necessarily *other* services, for all Medicare eligibles who have "countable" incomes below about $470 per month and liquid assets below $4,000. Of course, disabled and aged people who also meet the state's *regular* Medicaid eligibility rules would also get coverage of those other Medicaid services not covered at all by Medicare. This special feature is called the Qualified Medicare Buy-In ("QMB"), and the monthly income level for it will increase each year. (See final section of book and note 1 in SSDI section for further discussion of this point.)

Where SSI Recipients Apply for Medicaid, by State

"1634" States Where SSI Recipients "Automatically" Receive Medicaid

Alabama	Louisiana	Pennsylvania
Arizona	Maine	Rhode Island
Arkansas	Maryland	South Carolina
California	Massachusetts	South Dakota
Colorado	Michigan	Tennessee
Delaware	Mississippi	Texas
District of Columbia	Montana	Vermont
Florida	New Jersey	Washington
Georgia	New Mexico	West Virginia
Iowa	New York	Wisconsin
Kentucky		

"Title XVI" States Where SSI Recipients Get Medicaid by Showing Proof of SSI Eligibility to Welfare Office

Alaska	Nevada	Utah
Idaho	Oregon	Wyoming
Kansas		

"209(b)" States Where SSI Recipients Must Apply Separately for Medicaid at Welfare Office, Because Medicaid Rules Are Stricter than SSI Rules (in practice, though, virtually all SSI recipients will qualify for Medicaid as well)

Connecticut	Missouri	North Dakota
Hawaii	Nebraska	Ohio
Illinois	New Hampshire	Oklahoma
Indiana	North Carolina	Virginia
Minnesota		

Source: Author's personal files, updated by conversations with staff of the Health Care Financing Administration (HCFA), U.S. Department of Health and Human Services (HHS), as of mid-1989.

medical definition of disability[6] and was also financially eligible during
that period. Thus, it is *not* automatic. SSI applicants and recipients—
even in "1634" states—must apply for retroactive Medicaid *at the
local welfare office*. Because SSI eligibility determinations sometimes
take weeks or months, those who need retroactive Medicaid must file a
"pended" retroactive application *before or as soon as* they apply for
SSI.

· SSI applicants and recipients in "Title XVI" and "209(b)" states need
  to file "pended" applications for both retroactive and ongoing Medicaid
  at the local welfare office *before or as soon as* they apply for SSI,
  because if they wait for their SSI eligibility determinations (which
  sometimes take months), it may then be *too late* to apply to welfare for
  Medicaid (even under the retroactive provision).
· Even in "1634" states which "automatically" give Medicaid to SSI
  recipients, newly eligible SSI recipients may not receive their Medicaid
  cards in the mail for several weeks; if they need medical care right
  away, however, they can get manually issued Medicaid cards by
  reporting to the local welfare office with proof of their SSI eligibility.
· Some states and localities "station" their Medicaid eligibility workers
  at those area hospitals which tend to treat many uninsured patients.
  Many hospitals have their own specialized "financial counselors" or
  "charity care coordinators" in the business or registration office who
  can assist with and help file a patient's Medicaid application; otherwise,
  hospitals may designate one of the credit, finance, or billing clerks to
  assist with Medicaid applications. These workers are almost always
  skilled only in simple Medicaid eligibility. They will not know specialized, complex, unusual, or alternate provisions (such as those of
  SSI or AFDC) to acquire eligibility.
· Applicants should bring items shown in appendix E.
· Apply *at once*—do not delay applying to gather documents and verifications; it could mean loss of benefits. Supporting documents can be
  assembled later, if necessary.
· Another person can assist or apply for incapacitated persons; this
  includes relatives, friends, social workers, or other advocates.

6. This means that advocates must be vigilant to make sure doctors filling out SSDI/SSI and
Medicaid medical application forms have been careful enough to specify a "date of onset" of
the disability sufficiently early to cover the patient as "disabled"—and hence eligible for
Medicaid—for medical care during the retroactive 3 months. Unfortunately, doctors and even
applicants often thoughtlessly enter the current date or the date the patient first sought treatment, which can thereby undermine the application.

Detailed Spend Down Example

John's state has a one-person monthly Medicaid income eligibility level of $377 and it determines eligibility on a 6-month basis. Although the SSI monthly income level is $386, John's state pays an additional State Supplementary Payment (SSP) of $15, making the combined SSI/SSP level $401.[a] Each month John receives $600 from SSDI, and $299 gross from a part-time job. He pays a $60 monthly premium for a private health insurance policy which covers 80% of all medical care with no deductible. Since he has been on SSDI for less than 2 years, John does not yet receive Medicare.

On January 1, John applies for Medicaid. This is how the Medicaid eligibility worker computes his case:

$600 SSDI
−$20 general income disregard
$580 "countable" unearned income.

$299 gross earnings
−$65 earnings disregard[b]
$234 ÷ 2 =
$117 "countable" earned income.

$580 "countable" unearned income
+$117 "countable" earned income
$697 total monthly "countable" income.

$697 total monthly "countable" income
−$377 state eligibility level monthly
$320 monthly "excess income"
×6 number of months in state eligibility time period
$1,926 "excess income" for total 6-month state eligibility time period
−$360 (6 × $60), John's health insurance premium over 6 months[c]
$1,566 net remaining "excess income" that must be incurred on medical bills.

[a]Because of a complex formula in the Medicaid law, the Medicaid-only eligibility level to which applicants must spend down can sometimes be even lower than the SSI or SSI/SSP level.
[b]Note that SSI income disregards are used in this case, because the applicant is applying as disabled. For families and children, the AFDC income disregards would be used. See note 3 for "209(b)" states.
[c]Projected premiums for Medicare and private health insurance can be deducted for "spend down" purposes.

On January 2, John's Medicaid eligibility worker gives him a notice summarizing the above computations, denying him Medicaid for the time being, but telling him to return for a Medicaid card if his medical bills *incurred* (not necessarily *paid*) before June 30 (the end of the 6-month eligibility time period) equal $1,566. He cannot, however, get credit for bills paid, or expected to be paid, by his health insurance.

On January 3, John pays cash for $100 worth of prescriptions (which his health plan does not cover). From January 4 through 8, John goes into the hospital, running up a hospital bill and assorted other bills from various doctors. Because he needs a Medicaid card right away to pay for expensive prescriptions and home health care which his doctors ordered at discharge, John does not wait to receive his hospital and doctor bills by routine mail. Instead, he goes to the hospital and doctors' billing offices and has the staff make up interim bills while he waits, even if they have to be handwritten notes. He then takes the bills to the Medicaid eligibility worker (along with the "excess income" notification he got earlier and the forms or pamphlet from his health insurance plan showing its deductible and coverage/payment schedule).

This is how the eligibility worker will now compute John's case:[d]

$1,566 initial "excess income"
−$100 prescription paid for Jan. 3
$1,466 remaining "excess income" after Jan. 3
−$1,000 hospital charges for Jan. 4 (John's 20%; full charge is $5,000)
$466 subtotal.

$466
−$300 doctors' charges for Jan. 4 (John's 20%; full charge is $1,500)
$166 remaining "excess income" after Jan. 4.

$500 hospital charges for Jan. 5 (John's 20%; full charge is $2,500)
+$150 doctors' charges for Jan. 5 (John's 20%; full charge is $750)
$650 total charges for Jan. 5
−$166 John's remaining liability
$484 remaing Jan. 5th charges, to be covered by Medicaid.

[d]Where a Medicaid spend down applicant has Medicare or other insurance, the more accommodating states or eligibility workers will compute eligibility using *expected* rates of payment from the other insurance, based on the plan brochure; more rigid states or eligibility workers, however, will refuse to complete the computation until they see what the insurance *actually* pays—and since this takes months, the applicant goes without a Medicaid card until then.

John becomes eligible on January 5, being liable for $166 worth of care on that day, with Medicaid paying the balance of charges not covered by the insurance on that day and succeeding days until June 30. John is therefore given Medicaid for the period January 5–June 30. Out of John's total hospital and doctor bills for January 4–January 8, his private insurance will pay 80%, John will be liable for $1,466 out of his 20% share, and Medicaid will pay remaining costs.

Of course, this whole process will have to be repeated for the new 6-month eligibility period beginning July 1, when John will *again* have "excess income."

Note that Medicaid will *not* pay the $1,566 in bills which John used to "spend down" to the Medicaid level. The $1,566 is "excess income" which Medicaid expects—but does not *require*—John to pay on his own (the drug store, hospitals, and doctors, however, *will* attempt to require John to pay what he owes them). The drug store, of course, actually succeeded in requiring John to pay, since drug stores simply do not dispense prescriptions to anyone without money or an approved charge plan; the hospitals and doctors, on the other hand, do not have this advantage. Instead, they will have to bill John or attempt some collection action against him.

Even so, John still may not have to pay the bills. For one thing, he can ask the hospital and doctors to forgive his liability by accepting him as a Hill-Burton or charity patient. In addition, the actual amount of John's spend down liability will not be clear to the hospital or doctors' billing staffs. This is because *some* private health insurance plans and *all* Medicaid programs enjoy "discounts" off the face amounts of hospital bills (and even doctors' bills). Thus, if an unpaid deficit on the face amount of a bill remains after the discounted Medicaid payment is made, the billing staff will not necessarily know how much of the deficit results from the Medicaid discounting and how much from the patient's unpaid spend down liability. As a result, it is quite possible that the spend down liability amount will be mistakenly written off as part of the Medicaid discounting.

Source: Prepared by the author as a simplified amalgam of the several hundred spend down eligibility determinations in which he has participated.

4. Appeal Rights
- Every state has a system for a supervisory conference, a fair hearing, a review by the state director, and, finally, state or federal court action. Objections made within 10 days of each adverse decision will usually temporarily block termination or reduction of benefits; otherwise, the time limit is 60 days for appealing each adverse decision.
- SSI appeals provisions govern where SSI application has functioned simultaneously as Medicaid application.
- Hospitalized Medicaid patients dissatisfied with the quality of their care or with the hospital's discharge or placement arrangements should appeal *at once* to the Peer Review Organization serving their area (see appendix L). Pre-discharge complaints will delay and possibly (if upheld) cancel any poorly planned discharge and force the hospital to make adequate post-discharge housing arrangements for those who need them.

5. Additional Information and Special Problems
- Anyone applying for Medicaid who has not yet started to receive SSI or Social Security should be sure to apply for General Assistance while at the welfare office.
- Programs vary widely. Large industrial states have the most liberal rules; rural and southern states are the most restrictive (13 states do not even allow "spend down" for those with income initially above the eligibility level).
- Many newly disabled persons get Medicaid through SSI eligibility (see SSI section), because SSI payments can start *right away*. *Regular* Social Security disability benefits (that is, SSDI, which is based on one's work earnings record) have a 5-month waiting period. *Most* persons' SSDI awards will turn out, after the 5-month waiting period, to be *above the SSI income level* (because, while the SSI income level is $386, the average SSDI award is about $550). This means that, after the first 5 months, most disabled people *lose Medicaid* based on SSI status. The way to reestablish Medicaid coverage is through the "spend down," available in most—but not all—states. Usually, one or two days of hospitalization produces enough *incurred* (but not necessarily *paid*) medical bills to "spend down" to the Medicaid level, and eligibility reestablished this way can last for the rest of the state's eligibility time period (see Detailed Spend Down Example).
- Conversely, where states place an SSI recipient on Medicaid, oversight, high workloads, or computer systems can allow the recipient to remain

on Medicaid for 6 months, a year, or more; thus is neglected the fact
that after the 5-month SSDI waiting period, such persons' SSDI awards
might well raise them above the SSI level. This should render them
ineligible for Medicaid *as SSI recipients;* however, because of the
system inadequacies, it does not. Thus, ex-SSI recipients can receive
many months of Medicaid to which they are not properly entitled. Of
course, in these cases, such accidental Medicaid beneficiaries are
supposed to report such errors to the welfare office, even though it will
mean termination from Medicaid (with no alternate realistic way to
reacquire it in many states). However, where welfare offices do discover such errors, there are few meaningful penalties they can impose,
as future medical care can hardly be denied to continuing Medicaid-
eligibles, and because no non-federal claimant (even welfare offices)
can legally garnish SSI or SSDI checks.

· Some states, at their own expense, give "General Medical Assistance"
identical to Medicaid to poor persons who do *not* meet the SSDI/SSI
definition of disability, or who do not fit into one of the other federally
covered categories (such as over age 65, under age 7, certain other
children, pregnant women, or AFDC-type families). Some offer a
"watered down" medical assistance to these people (such as treatment
only in public hospitals and clinics, or only as authorized on a funds-
available, bill-by-bill basis). The most rural, conservative areas grant
little or no coverage (see General Assistance section and
appendix C).

· The "spend down" of *incurred* (but not necessarily *paid*) bills to the
Medicaid eligibility level only applies to excess income—*not to excess
assets.* Those with excess assets can only become eligible on the day
after they *actually expend* their excess assets on medical care or modest
living expenses. Anyone who gives away, sells for less than market
value, or squanders excess assets will be found ineligible for Medicaid.

· Generally, participation by medical care providers in Medicaid is
voluntary. While almost all hospitals, clinics, pharmacies, home health
agencies, and hospices participate in their state's Medicaid program,
many (in some areas, *most*) physicians and other single practitioners
refuse to do so—usually because of low Medicaid fee schedules and the
requirement that they accept the Medicaid rate as full payment. Therefore, many Medicaid patients need help from the welfare office, the
health department, medical societies, social workers, and hospitals in
locating Medicaid-participating physicians. Some welfare offices have
lists of participating doctors. However, advocates should bear in mind

that any hospital which *ever* accepted Hill-Burton funds (even those which no longer must give free care) are required to *compel* staff physicians to participate in Medicaid (even if such doctors ordinarily refuse to do so) in order to treat Medicaid patients for inpatient, outpatient department, or emergency room care. Moreover, groups in several New England states have proposed general medical licensure laws *requiring* all doctors to participate in Medicaid and to accept its fee schedule. See appendix G–2 for groups advocating this approach in your state.

· Federal law requires that those Medicaid patients whose eligibility arose from SSI or SSP receipt, and who later lose SSI or SSP because of SSDI cost-of-living increases, will *retain Medicaid as if they were still SSI/SSP recipients.*

Hill-Burton, Private Hospital Charity Care, and Public Hospitals and Clinics

The U.S. Public Health Service's "Hill-Burton" program gives grants and guarantees loans for hospital construction, renovation, and expansion. Hospitals which receive this help—even private, non-charity hospitals—are required to grant free or partially free hospitalization to low-income persons who are not completely covered by health insurance, Medicare, or Medicaid.

Not all hospitals have Hill-Burton—only those which have received federal construction help are required to participate. However, all publicly owned or operated hospitals—and even some private, non-charity hospitals—have some sort of in-house, charity, bill write-off program for those with no way to pay who meet income (and, sometimes, asset) guidelines. In addition, a variety of federal, state, local, and private philanthropic health agencies finance free or reduced-fee health clinics, which are typically run by local health departments or nonprofit agencies.

1. Eligibility

- Generally those with income below the federal poverty level (in 1990, about $522 for one person monthly) are fully eligible, with partial bill reductions sometimes available on a sliding scale as income rises above that level. Income and asset levels vary from state to state, locality to locality, and even health program to health program.
- All Hill-Burton facilities give free care to those with incomes up to the poverty level; many, however, also take the federally offered option of also giving free care to those with incomes up to *twice* the poverty level (about $1,045 monthly in 1990).
- For those becoming eligible for Medicaid via a "spend down" (see Medicaid section), Hill-Burton and hospital charity bill write-offs can cover the portion of a hospital's bill which would otherwise be the patient's liability.
- Services are available to *all* needy residents, not just to those found "disabled."

· Hill-Burton programs have no *assets* eligibility level and no income disregards; other programs' assets and income disregard policies vary.
· Hospital Hill-Burton and charity programs, as well as many local low-income clinics, require an applicant to apply for and follow through on Medicaid or other public medical assistance: eligibility is then granted only to those found ineligible for complete Medicaid coverage of their bills.

2. Benefits

· Free or reduced-fee inpatient hospital, low-income health clinic, and (depending on facility) outpatient department and emergency room services.
· Free or reduced-fee outpatient prescription drugs at many clinics and some hospital outpatient departments (drugs "to go" are rarely dispensed by hospital emergency room or inpatient treatment programs).
· At all Hill-Burton hospitals and clinics (even those no longer offering free care) the facility *must:*
  · admit otherwise qualified area residents even if they do not have a personal doctor with admitting privileges
  · require staff doctors to accept Medicare or Medicaid from admitted patients who have such coverage
  · treat in the emergency room, and, if medically necessary, admit to inpatient care, *any* patient needing emergency care, without regard to insurance coverage, ability to pay, Medicare/Medicaid status or lack of a personal physician with staff privileges
  · not demand advance deposits from Hill-Burton, Medicare, or Medicaid patients, even for "elective" admissions
  · not demand advance deposits from *any* needy, uncovered patient if a reasonable installment payment plan is agreed to by the patient, even for "elective" admission

3. How and Where to Apply

· If such a person exists, apply with the designated "Hill-Burton coordinator," "charity care counselor," or "financial counselor"; otherwise, you may have to question several credit or billing clerks before you locate the person authorized to grant free Hill-Burton or charity care. It may be the manager of the credit or billing office. But in every hospital, *someone* has authority to forgive or reduce bills; be persistent.
· Generally, hospitals and clinics require the submission of verifications shown in appendix E.

· Hill-Burton has written rules and application forms.
· Some hospital charity programs and local low-income clinics may have written rules and application forms; however, if they do not, the decision to grant charity care may be made informally or even verbally by the hospital or clinic credit, billing, or registration director.
· If a patient waits to receive the hospital bill or a Medicaid eligibility determination via "spend down" (which can occur months after discharge), he or she can still apply for Hill-Burton, as there is no time limit on its applications. Obviously, however, it makes most sense to apply at the time of hospitalization, particularly because other programs *are* likely to have time limits.

4. Appeal Rights

· Those dissatisfied with Hill-Burton eligibility decisions or hospital compliance with other Hill-Burton rules can appeal by contacting the regional offices of the U.S. Department of Health and Human Services (HHS) listed in appendix F. State health departments handle these complaints in California, Minnesota, Montana, Ohio, South Dakota, and Vermont. The Hill-Burton program maintains a complaint hotline; call (800) 638-0742; (800) 492-0359 in Maryland.
· Decisions about eligibility for Hill-Burton or hospital charity care can be appealed *informally* to the credit, billing, or finance manager; to the hospital vice president for finance; to the hospital director or president; and finally, the hospital board.
· Appeal rights for local low-income health clinics vary enormously. If the facility has received a Hill-Burton grant, then those appeal provisions apply. Otherwise, such facilities typically have a "patient's bill of rights" or similar document setting forth appeal rights. Clinics run by local and state government bodies may also have their own appeal rules.

5. Additional Information and Special Problems

· Hill-Burton and most hospital charity programs only cover inpatient hospital bills—*not* doctors' bills. Some hospitals do not permit use of Hill-Burton for outpatient department or emergency room bills.
· If a hospital bill has been forgiven or reduced by Hill-Burton or a hospital charity program, one must apply *separately* to the doctor's billing office (usually in another building) to request a write-off of the accompanying doctor's bill. (Doctors are *not* required to do this, but many do so as a gesture of good-will for those accepted by the hospital.)

- Hospital social workers can offer information, referral, and moral support for those seeking free care—*but they do not determine eligibility.* Do not make the error of assuming they will "handle it" based on conversations with or promises from them: the decision-makers are in the credit, billing, or registration office.
- Even if accepted for Hill-Burton or charity care, one may still receive a bill because of paperwork errors or computer problems. *Get the decision in writing;* if staff will not do so, make note of staff member's name, title, office, and date for one's own future protection.
- Lists of hospitals subject to Hill-Burton requirements are available from regional offices of HHS (see appendix F) and from some state and local health departments.

FOR FURTHER INFORMATION . . .

A good recent overview of the Hill-Burton, state-local, and hospital-based care for indigents is *Too Poor To Be Sick,* by Patricia Butler, available from the American Public Health Association for $17.50. An exhaustive review of Hill-Burton program requirements, *The Right To Health Care,* by Armin Freifield (order no. 41,900; $15.00), is available from the National Clearinghouse for Legal Services. See appendix G–1 for ordering addresses.

Mental Health and Substance Abuse Programs

All states and most localities have publicly funded free or reduced-fee mental health and substance abuse programs, financed with a combination of federal, state, and local funds. The state or local health department runs these programs, usually through subsidiary mental health, mental hospital, alcoholism, or drug abuse agencies.

1. Eligibility

- Coverage is given for free services—or with small co-payments—to those on welfare, SSI, or Medicaid, or those who have low income or none at all.
- Reduced-fee services are given to those with higher incomes, usually on a sliding-scale basis. State income levels vary.
- Services are available to *all* needy residents (that is, it is not limited only to those found "disabled").
- Most localities permit cars and *lived-in* homes; liquid asset levels vary.
- Better-off applicants will have to pay the full cost of care or be referred to private medical providers.
- Because of free or sliding-scale fee schedules and what amounts to "open admission" for those who need emergency treatment, these programs' eligibility rules can be *significantly more liberal than* those of Medicaid.

2. Benefits

- Hospitalization in state or local mental hospitals.
- Individual or group therapy.
- "Significant other" counseling.
- Psychoactive and anti-depressant medications.
- Alcohol and drug detoxification and treatment.
- Methadone programs.
- Crisis interventions, commitments, hotlines, etc.
- Home mental health care in some areas.
- Often, *free physical health care* for inpatients in state or local mental

hospitals or inpatient detoxification programs (even if they have no Medicaid or other way to pay).

3. How and Where to Apply
- Apply at intake or registration or admissions office of mental health center, state or local mental hospital or drug/alcohol facility.
- Bring items shown for "Hospitals" in appendix E.

4. Appeal Rights
- These vary. Most states and localities have a "patient's bill of rights" or similar written standards, setting forth the applicant's or patient's appeal and grievance rights.

5. Additional Information and Special Problems
- Program rules and availability of services vary enormously.
- Because of the relationship between IV drug abuse and much HIV infection, some areas' drug programs go *far beyond* simple detoxification treatment and offer partial or complete physical health care packages—this might be particularly useful for those not eligible for Medicaid.
- Under special waivers obtained by a few states and localities, *more liberal* Medicaid eligibility and coverage packages are offered for those in certain state or local substance abuse programs (this would permit, therefore, Medicaid coverage of non-detoxification-related medical care).

Housing and Mortgage Delinquency Programs

Public Housing and Rental Assistance

With federal funding, many state, city, or county housing departments run a variety of housing programs for low-income persons, with special projects or units set aside for the aged and disabled. All of these programs generally charge rents of 30% of tenants' adjusted gross income (including SSI and welfare).

· Public housing projects for low-income families are what most people think of as "low-income housing." The stereotype is generally accurate: they are inhabited by welfare mothers, they are poorly maintained and dangerous, but they nonetheless have long waiting lists. Generally, they are of little use or interest to most childless PWAs.

· "Senior citizens' housing" projects—some public, some private—are perceived as much less unpleasant by the general public, but these too are low-income projects. Less well known, however, is the fact that these projects are often meant for the *disabled* as well as for the aged. Disability benefits from SSDI, SSI, Medicaid, the VA, the civil service, and even from General Assistance can qualify one for these projects. The waiting lists are long, but not nearly so long as those for "welfare mother" public housing projects.

· Other federally aided housing for the disabled and aged is usually in private projects. It consists of two types, the first being particular apartments or whole buildings whose residents receive rental subsidies or inexpensive rents on some other basis. The other type uses "portable" certificates and vouchers for rental subsidy, which qualified holders can present to any participating landlord. The waiting lists for both variations of this program are very long; however, the separate waiting lists for the aged and disabled are far shorter than those for the general public.

· Priority within the waiting lists for programs described above is granted to disabled or aged persons who are presently paying more than 50% of their adjusted gross incomes for housing, who have been displaced by urban renewal and similar programs, or who live in housing found to be substandard.

· Some states and localities fund their own counterparts to federally aided programs, complete with the "fixed" subsidized units and "portable" subsidy certificates and vouchers. Again, these programs have separate and shorter waiting lists for the disabled and aged.

· Eligibility under these programs is generally limited to those with incomes below 80% of the area's median (or, in some cases, 50%); in addition, local agencies can (but not all do) establish an *assets* test as well. (Note that while *most* needs-based programs exclude a *lived-in* home as an asset, housing programs can arguably exclude such home-owners on the grounds that such a home negates their "need" for housing, absent unusual circumstances.)

· Apply at state, city, or county housing agency, bringing items shown in appendix E. For *some* public projects, and for *many* private units or projects, applications, waiting list numbers, and unit assignments are handled *at the rental office of the particular project*. Ask the public housing agency for a list of projects which have independent applica-tion procedures or waiting lists.

· Where private developers, in order to get zoning clearances, have committed themselves to offering inexpensive rents to low or moderate income persons in some of their rental units, *these projects may not be known to and listed by the housing agency*. Instead, projects offering these inexpensive rents might only be listed by the city or county zoning or planning office.

· Anyone with a grievance, such as being denied eligibility, threatened with eviction, dissatisfied with rent amount or proposed rent increase, assessed for "overpayments" or repair/damage costs, denied return of deposit, transferred to an unacceptable unit, dissatisfied with waiting list or priority category or unit placement, or who otherwise has a grievance against program decisions, may request a conference with the project manager, or if still dissatisfied, a "hearing" or "review" within a "reasonable time." In most localities this means within 10 days of the agency's notification of an action, particularly if the applicant or resident wishes to prevent loss of ongoing benefits. The "hearing" or "review" must be conducted by an impartial referee or a board uninvolved with the program decision, and the applicant or resident must be given a prompt, written decision. For proposed evictions, housing agencies may, with HUD approval, instead utilize the existing landlord/tenant legal processes of the state's court system as an alternative to the required grievance process. Further appeals can then be taken to state or federal courts.

· Independent and otherwise legal actions by *private* project management are not strictly grievable.

· Because of recent publicity about drug-related violence in public housing projects, HUD is now (as of late 1989) considering legislation and regulations to bar admission, and swiftly to evict, those who (or whose household members) are believed to represent immediate dangers to tenants' health and safety. Such new rules could foreshorten, or even negate, housing program grievance/appeals procedures or even general state landlord/tenant court hearings, depending upon the success of legal challenges by tenant legal advocacy groups. Because of the connection between drug use and much HIV infection, development of this issue should be followed by PWA benefits advocates.

· See the following section concerning the availability of housing in board and care homes.

FOR FURTHER INFORMATION . . .

Because there is such a variety of federal (not to mention state and local) public housing and rental assistance programs, it is difficult to summarize their provisions in a uniform, coherent outline. A detailed *Introduction to HUD-Subsidized Housing Programs* by Fred Fuchs (order no. 33,843–B; $11.50) and an update in the March 1988 issue of *Clearinghouse Review* ($6.00) are available from the National Clearinghouse for Legal Services (see appendix G–1 for ordering address).

Mortgage Delinquency Programs

A variety of federal laws, regulations, and policies can prevent foreclosures and otherwise secure relief for those with delinquent home mortgages insured by the Federal Housing Administration (FHA), the Department of Housing and Urban Development (HUD), and the Department of Veterans Affairs (VA). These rights generally exceed those available under conventional and state-insured, -guaranteed, and -subsidized mortgages. The federal mortgage delinquency provisions are set forth in appendix I, an excerpt from *Foreclosure Prevention Programs Available to Homeowners with Governmentally Insured Mortgages* by Robert F. Gillett. PWAs and advocates confronting delinquencies should secure review of this material by staff or volunteers who are attorneys, bankers, or realtors with technical expertise in mortgage and other real estate matters.

In addition, a number of mortgage documents themselves—or their issuing financial institutions—have provisions setting forth remedies for the homeowner's delinquency due to disability or death. Even more commonly, mortgages may be supplemented by credit life (and even disability) insurance policies offering loan payoff or other subsidies or remedies. Sometimes lenders take out such policies for all or much of their home mortgage loan portfolio—and the homeowner may not necessarily know of such protection. Finally, state and local regulations for *their* publicly financed, insured, guaranteed, or underwritten home mortgages—as well as general state regulations for banks and lending institutions—may provide some relief approaching that available at the federal level. Again, attorneys, bankers, or realtors with technical expertise in local real estate/mortgage procedures should be consulted.

Board and Care Homes

Almost all states have even higher State Supplementary Payments (SSPs), which they add to the "living independently" SSI or SSI/SSP level, for needy disabled persons living in "board and care homes." Board and care homes are publicly or privately operated group residences which provide nonprofessional, nonmedical, personal assistance and meals and lodging to two or more unrelated aged or disabled adults. They are often loosely—and inaccurately—called "nursing homes" by the lay public, but actually they offer supervised group home care at a "sub-medical" level, that is, below the level of medical care provided in skilled nursing facilities (SNFs) and intermediate care facilities (ICFs). Eligibility, benefits, appeals, and other facets of SSPs for board and care homes are discussed in the chapter on "State Supplementary Payments (SSPs)."

· This additional SSP amount is added to the basic SSI levels of disabled persons on the theory that it will cost them more to rent room and board in a group home specifically catering to the disabled. Thus, those living in such homes have, in effect, a special "extra high" SSI eligibility level applied to their cases (see appendix B) to pay their rents if they have insufficient SSDI or other non-welfare-type income with which to do so.

· Local welfare, health, and licensure staff do *not* use or even know the national, generic term "board and care home." Instead, state and local staff use their own local bureaucratic terms for these places: "adult," "boarding," "community," "residential," "foster," "congregate," "group," "project," "supervised," "special," "rest," "aged," "domiciliary," and "family" homes.

· The SSP is sometimes paid by Social Security, sometimes by the welfare office (see appendix B). However, in all cases, some sort of placement authorization by the "adult services," "nursing home," or "level of care determination" division of the welfare office is necessary. These "placement authorizations" can be appealed as can any other welfare program decision (see appeals discussions in Medicaid section).

- Eligibility for a board and care home SSP also confers Medicaid eligibility.
- Board and care homes usually must meet relatively simple health department licensure rules; as a result, not only localities, but also small nonprofit groups and even private homeowners operate board and care homes, with much of their "rent" derived from the increased SSPs payable to needy disabled residents.
- Residents with sufficient incomes from SSDI or other non-welfare-type sources, of course, simply pay their own rents as would any other private tenant.
- Board and care home residents may not be required to pay their entire incomes for room and board; all states or localities set rent ceilings and *minimum* amounts residents retain as "personal needs allowances" (at *least* $30 monthly, but often quite more) for entertainment, transportation, clothing, laundry, toiletries, gifts, and any other ordinary non-room-and-board expenses. Usually, states permit board and care home operators to charge *less* than the state-set rate, if they wish, and thereby permit residents to retain more of their income.
- In some areas, local gay and AIDS-related groups run board and care homes for needy residents with AIDS, and the residents can thereby qualify for increased SSPs.
- Details about state board and care SSPs are provided in appendix B.
- In a number of areas, mental health, mental retardation, health department, and other public and private charity funds as well as social services block grants are used to subsidize board and care home operating costs. This means that not *all* costs would be covered by high rents paid with specialized board and care SSPs (if residents are needy). Where a home is financed in this way residents would not be eligible for board and care SSPs; instead they would merely be eligible (if needy) for SSI and whatever *general* SSP is available in the state (which they would then use to pay whatever rent such a subsidized home would charge them).
- HIV-infected "boarder babies" now in medical institutions can become eligible for SSI and an SSP for board and care—and thus can be cared for in home-like group residences rather than in inappropriate hospitals (see discussion of foster care in AFDC section).
- Across the U.S., many thousands of board and care homes—including the few established in recent years by gay and AIDS-related groups—have not pursued licensure with state authorities, because of ignorance of these programs, reluctance to endure the bureaucratic processing, or

fear that facilities simply cannot meet standards. However, advocates should reconsider carefully nonparticipation: residents thus lose the potential for significantly higher board and care SSP incomes (and thereby Medicaid eligibility, which might not be possible for them otherwise). To this end, public agencies are increasingly helpful in assisting facilities to qualify for licensure, often providing funding and training. Moreover, in most states, operation of unlicensed board and care homes is *illegal* and subject to administrative, civil, and even criminal penalties.

· These programs are operated by some unit of the health or welfare department and can be located in the government sections of the phone book under subsections such as "Welfare Department—Adult Services," "Health Department—Nursing Home Licenses," or "Licenses—Boarding Houses."

· The Health Resources and Services Administration (HRSA) in HHS' Public Health Service makes AIDS services demonstration project grants, which can include board and care home services as part of an overall PWA health service program. It also makes AIDS services planning grants, which can include planning and startup costs for board and care homes, again, when they are to be part of an overall PWA health program. Section 301 of the Public Health Service Act, as amended by Public Laws 100–202 and 100–436, authorizes these programs. Contact Richard Schulman, Room 9A05 HRSA, 5600 Fishers Lane, Rockville, MD 20857, (301) 443–0652, for details.

· HRSA also makes grants *specifically* for construction and renovation of PWA board and care homes where the supervised residential placement is to be part of a patient care plan written and monitored by a physician *or* a PWA health/social service organization. Contact Katherine Buckner, Room 11A10 HRSA, 5600 Fishers Lane, Rockville, MD 20857, (301) 443–0271, for details.

· Other sources for financing PWA board and care homes are set forth in works by these authors cited in the bibliography: Capitman, Chen, and Coopers, Department of Housing and Urban Development, Harmon, Health Resources and Services Administration, Joe, Ponce, Reisacher, Reschovsky, and Stone.

· Local government and neighborhood opposition to PWA group homes, and how to overcome it, is discussed by Milstein, Pepper, and Stiehl.

· General board and care issues are addressed by Cohen, Jameson, Komlos-Hrobsky, Laudicina, McCormack, Smith, and Wetch.

Low Income Home Energy Assistance (LIHEA)

Low Income Home Energy Assistance is a federal-state welfare program which pays heating—and, in some cases, cooling—costs for low-income persons.

1. Eligibility
- States can elect to use an income eligibility level equal to 150% of the poverty level (about $783 monthly in 1990) or 60% of that state's median income level.
- Otherwise, states can limit eligibility to those on SSI, AFDC, or Food Stamps, or who have incomes below 110% of the poverty level (about $574 monthly in 1990).
- States do not count a *lived-in* home or modest automobile in figuring eligibility.
- A few states have liquid asset eligibility levels similar to those of SSI ($2,000) or AFDC ($1,500).
- Most states disregard at least some of disabled persons' income if it is spent on medical expenses.

2. Benefits
- Payment of some or all of home heating costs such as gas, oil, coal, electricity, and wood bills.
- In some states, payment of some or all home air conditioning costs such as electricity or gas bills.
- In some states, payment or provision of some or all of heating or air conditioning equipment or repair costs.
- In most states, some costs of home weatherization (such as caulking and storm windows).
- In some states, payment of some or all costs attributable to heating or air conditioning costs, even if these are included in the applicant's overall rental payment.
- Shortages of funds mean that, in most states, only a part of the applicant's energy costs can be covered.

3. How and Where to Apply

· In some states, one applies for Low Income Home Energy Assistance at the welfare office, while in others applications are made at a separate energy office; in all cases, the welfare office will know where to apply (see city or county section of phone book).
· Bring items shown in appendix E.

4. Appeal Rights

· Every state has a system for a supervisory conference, a fair hearing, a review by the state director, and, finally, state or federal court action. Objections made within 10 days of each adverse decision will usually temporarily block termination or reduction of benefits; otherwise, the time limit is 30 days for appealing each adverse decision.

5. Additional Information and Special Problems

· Low Income Home Energy Assistance varies enormously from state to state, and funds are severely limited.
· In some areas, coverage of air conditioning/air purification costs may require a doctor's note attesting to medical necessity (for reasons such as difficulty breathing or danger of infection).
· In some areas, utilities administer charity funds, or otherwise have programs to discount or forgive utility bills, particularly for the low-income elderly or disabled. The Low Income Home Energy Assistance staff, or the utilities themselves, will know of such programs.
· In many areas, the Emergency Assistance program will pay utility arrears for those facing imminent cutoff and will often pay reconnection or deposit charges, as well as arrears, for those whose service has already been cut off.
· Those facing imminent cutoff can often get a delay by contacting the utility and discussing a payment schedule, pointing out pending benefits (such as SSDI, SSI, Emergency Assistance, welfare, or Low Income Home Energy Assistance), explaining nonpayment due to extended hospitalization, and finally, by negotiating some sort of bill reduction.
· Some local laws or utilities' own policies bar cutoff of heating sources during winter months as a matter of health and public relations.

Health and Life Insurance

Although health and life insurance coverage does not strictly fall within the realm of *public* benefits, some brief mention should be made of such coverage as it relates to public benefits for health and income. Retention of any employer-based life insurance coverage is a vital and obvious need for PWAs and PWARCs whose medical status requires their leaving full-time employment. And while retention of any employer-based *health* insurance may appear less crucial to such PWAs and PWARCs—given the common assumptions that Medicaid, Medicare, and other public health care will be readily available—the fact is that steps to retain or convert health insurance must *always* be considered when employment ends.

Such retention is vital because (1) not all PWARCs will be "disabled enough" to get Medicaid; (2) the lack of a Medicaid "spend down" in 13 states means that some PWAs and PWARCs will have incomes above SSI/Medicaid levels and thus be "too rich" for Medicaid; and (3) many PWAs and PWARCs who initially get Medicaid through SSI eligibility will lose SSI/Medicaid after the 5-month SSDI waiting period (if their SSDI awards turn out to be above the SSI level). In short, in states without "spend down," the receipt of SSDI, or other income which is initially above the SSI level, or which rises above it after 5 months, means *ineligibility for Medicaid.* Additionally, those few PWAs and PWARCs with adequate incomes will still find the cost of extending health insurance far less burdensome than large Medicaid "spend downs." As a result, extension of employer-based health insurance—as well as life insurance—should be carefully reviewed in every case where employment ceases.

Life Insurance

Obviously, PWAs and PWARCs are almost always unable to purchase individual life insurance policies. Where a previously purchased individual policy exists, all efforts should be made to meet premium payments and retain coverage—when and if it lapses, all chance of individual coverage ends forever.

Policies must be read with great care, as "grace period" and "reinstatement" rules can be quite complex and vary enormously from policy to policy. Even those who seem hopelessly delinquent in paying premiums might discover obscure provisions allowing them to "pay up" or "reinstate" an apparently lapsed policy.

Those who have been employed often have work-based life insurance coverage (in some cases, the employee may not even be aware of this; a check with the personnel or payroll office, though, can confirm the existence of coverage). *Life insurance coverage is almost always available for extension or conversion without a medical exam, "pre-existing condition" exclusion, or waiting period.* Of course, the ex-employee (or someone acting on his behalf) would have to undertake timely premium payments himself; moreover, these premiums might be higher than those previously paid by the employer.

Again, as with individual policies, some careful reading of the employer's master policy provisions may be necessary—especially in verifying whether apparently "lapsed" conversion/extension rights of those who appear "delinquent" have, in fact, finally been lost. Except when dealing with the largest employers, who have highly skilled employee benefits specialists, it may be necessary to contact the insurance broker who sold the policy to the employer, in order to review and possibly to salvage difficult or seemingly lapsed conversion/extension rights. (The clerical-level staff who handle employee benefits in small or even midsize firms may, unfortunately, not understand or know enough to provide expert guidance in more intricate or difficult cases.) Unlike the health insurance industry, life insurance matters are *not* subject to uniform federal laws; state regulation varies enormously and is often weak (see appendix K).

COLLECTING ON A LIFE INSURANCE POLICY WHILE STILL ALIVE
Until recently, it has been impossible for terminally ill persons to collect on their life insurance policies before their deaths, via loans, advances, or assignments. Recently, however, one firm has developed such a program, and it has proved beneficial to a number of PWAs. In essence, someone covered by a life insurance policy assigns ownership of the policy irrevocably to the firm and names it beneficiary, after securing legal consents from both the life insurance company and the previously named beneficiaries. The firm then pays the insured terminally ill person between 60% and 75% of the face amount of the policy, depending upon medically documented life expectancy, the amount of the policy, and other factors. The life insurance policy must be an *individual* one (not employer group), and it must have been in force for at least 2 years. (However, time under a previous group plan which is later converted to an individual

policy counts toward the 2-year minimum, and almost all group life plans are, in fact, so convertible.) The patient must have a life expectancy of 18 months or less, and the face policy amount must be at least $50,000—but these points are negotiable if the terminally ill person will accept lesser payments. Finally, an applicant for these payments must provide all medical, hospital, clinic, and insurance records to the firm. Further information is available from Living Benefits, Inc., at 6110 Seagull Lane, N.E., Suite 108, Albuquerque, New Mexico 87109. The telephone number is (800) 458–8790 or (505) 883–4799.

VETERANS' GROUP LIFE INSURANCE
Group life insurance policies of active-duty servicemen may be converted, without a medical exam, within 120 days after discharge (but as long as a year later in the case of total disability), to a 5-year term policy, which is not renewable. However, the term policy may *then*—again without medical exam—be converted to an individual policy through the Office of Servicemen's Group Life Insurance, at 213 Washington Street, Newark, NJ 07102. Details are available at VA offices. Also, all veterans with service-connected disabilities may take out inexpensive (sometimes even free) life insurance policies of up to $10,000—no matter how long after discharge and what their medical condition.

Health Insurance

EXTENDING BENEFITS WITH COBRA
The Consolidated Omnibus Budget Reconciliation Act of 1985 (COBRA) requires employers of 20 or more with group health insurance to allow those leaving employment to remain covered in the group plan (with the same benefit package) for up to 29 months *if they pay the full premiums themselves.* Employers must notify departing employees of this option in writing and explain payments and procedures required to exercise it. The employee generally is given 60 days after the date of the notice (rather than after the last day of work) to take the option and make premium payments—although premiums must be paid retroactively to the last day of employer-paid coverage. Parallel and longer extension protections are also available for dependents of ex-employees and those who have *lost* their status as dependents of employees (such as divorced spouses or children who reach majority).

COBRA also gives the ex-employee *conversion* rights (*after* the 29-month extension) to an individual health policy with the same insurer; the ex-employee is responsible for premium payments. Individual *conversion* policies may not impose a medical exam, a "preexisting condition" clause or a waiting period as a condition of coverage; however, premiums for *these* policies are likely to cost more than COBRA group coverage extensions, and their benefit/coverage packages are almost always more limited. For those without any other alternatives for medical coverage, however, conversion policies are an invaluable bargain.

In addition to federal COBRA continuation/conversion rights, a number of states also mandate health insurance extensions for former employees. While these state requirements are generally identical to or even less stringent than the federal COBRA rules, they can differ from COBRA in one vital particular: some apply to employer groups of less than 20 (which COBRA does not). And, of course, as with COBRA, the employee would have to begin premium payments himself, and where a conversion (as opposed to a *continuation*) option is invoked, the coverage package may be less extensive than under the employer plan itself, and premiums may be higher. Details about state requirements are available from state insurance commissioners or departments (see appendix K). States with health insurance continuation/conversion requirements include the following:

Arizona	Massachusetts	Oregon
Arkansas	Minnesota	Pennsylvania
California	Missouri	Rhode Island
Colorado	Montana	South Carolina
Connecticut	Nebraska	South Dakota
Florida	New Hampshire	Tennessee
Georgia	New Jersey	Texas
Illinois	New Mexico	Virginia
Iowa	New York	Washington
Kansas	North Carolina	West Virginia
Kentucky	Ohio	Wisconsin
Maine	Oklahoma	Wyoming
Maryland		

Even without the compulsion of COBRA, many employers *voluntarily* continue health and life insurance premium payments (often for considerable times) for those employees who are hospitalized or awaiting SSDI/SSI/Medicaid eligibility. These altruistic and patient employers need to be recognized and encouraged, as their continued financing of premiums not only can save an often needy PWA from having to pay, but they buy him or her that much more time later under COBRA. As weakening employees approach resignation from their jobs, or when their illness episodes result in decisions not to return to work, aggressive but diplomatic advocacy with employers should be brought to bear to induce this voluntary, continued payment of premiums. Many employers will readily do so, when asked, in order to allow employees time to secure Medicaid and other public benefits.

STATE-SPONSORED CATASTROPHIC HEALTH INSURANCE PROGRAMS
Several states operate or sponsor catastrophic health insurance programs—often for those who are otherwise "uninsurable"—for patients with extraordinarily high medical expenses. Plan provisions vary enormously: premiums may exceed those charged to the general public; there may be "preexisting condition" clauses or waiting periods; and there are almost always large deductibles. States with such programs are California, Idaho, Nevada, New Hampshire, New York, Oklahoma, Rhode Island, and South Dakota. In New Jersey the plan is only for children; a previously abandoned Minnesota program is now being planned for implementation. The Massachusetts Health Security Law already offers Medicaid-type benefits to disabled children and workers and the unemployed, as well as Hill-Burton-like free care for indigents in all hospitals in the state; by 1992, all state residents will be covered.

Information about these state catastrophic health insurance plans is available through the state insurance commissioner or department, usually in the respective state capitals. See appendix K.

STATE-SPONSORED "HIGH RISK" HEALTH INSURANCE POOLS
A number of other states operate or sponsor "high risk" health insurance pools for those who might otherwise be uninsurable, by requiring some or all health insurance companies operating in the state to participate jointly in covering such patients. Again, plans vary from state to state: premiums are higher than those for the general public; there may even be "preexisting condition" clauses or waiting periods; and there may be high deductibles or large coverage gaps. States with such programs are Connecticut, Florida, Illinois, Indiana, Iowa, Maine, Massachusetts, Minnesota, Montana, Nebraska, New Mexico, North Dakota, Oregon, Tennessee, Washington, and Wisconsin.[1]

Information about these state high risk health insurance pools is available through the state insurance commissioner or department. See appendix K.

1. Of these, the states which subsidize premiums for low- or moderate-income residents are: Indiana, Iowa, Maine, Minnesota, Nebraska, and Oregon.

Moreover, Maine and Wisconsin have short or no waiting periods for "preexisting conditions."

AARP HEALTH AND HOSPITALIZATION INSURANCE

The American Association of Retired Persons (AARP) markets to its *regular* members (those over age 50) an inexpensive "income-protection-during-hospitalization" insurance plan, for cash payable to a member for time in hospital. To enroll as a regular AARP member, send your name, address, birthdate, and $5 annual dues to:

American Association of Retired Persons (AARP)
Membership Processing Center
P.O. Box 199
Long Beach, CA 90801–9989

FOR FURTHER INFORMATION . . .

This section has only given the barest outline of the issues, options, and problems surrounding life and health insurance coverage for PWAs. More detailed guidance is contained in "The COBRA Continuation Options: Questions and Answers" in the April 1988 issue of *Clearinghouse Review* (available from the National Clearinghouse for Legal Affairs in Chicago, or in any good law library) and "Insurance and AIDS-Related Issues" in the *AIDS Practice Manual* (1988), available from National Gay Rights Advocates in San Francisco, or in any good law library. State laws mandating continuation or conversion of employer group health insurance plans are discussed further in Lawrence Bartlett and Judy Hoffman, *State Options for Improving Access to Care for the Uninsured,* a report commissioned by the American Association of Retired Persons (AARP) from Health Systems Research, Inc. in 1987. Addresses for ordering appear in appendix G–1.

Death, Taxes, Lawyers, and Special Medical and Disability Benefits

Death and Dying

PWAs in almost all states have the right to execute legal documents called "Living Wills," which instruct medical personnel and loved ones on the patient's choices regarding treatment. Orders concerning visitation when family and lover are at odds, "heroic measures," life sustaining equipment, respirators, artificial feeding, pain management, "do not resuscitate" codes, and many other decisions can thus be written in advance. In addition, either separately or as part of a "Living Will," a patient can extend a "Durable Power of Attorney" (different from ordinary powers of attorney, which usually only cover finances and may expire upon a patient's incapacity) to a trusted loved one for health care and all other major decisions when the patient is impaired. These documents should be drawn up by an attorney (see Free Legal Services subsection below). More detailed discussion of these and related issues is contained in National Gay Rights Advocates' *AIDS Practice Manual,* the American Association of Retired Persons' *A Matter of Choice: Planning Ahead for Health Care Decisions* (free), and Legal Counsel for the Elderly's *Decision-Making, Incapacity and the Elderly* ($34.95). See appendix G–1 for ordering information.

An organization which has taken an interest in individuals' death decisions is the Society for the Right to Die, 250 West 57th Street, Room 323, New York, NY 10107, telephone (212) 246–6973. (This organization will send preprinted "Living Will" and "Health Care Power of Attorney" forms to those who send a stamped, self-addressed, large business envelope.) The Hemlock Society, P.O. Box 11830, Eugene, OR 97440, telephone (503) 342–5748, provides information about painless dying and related issues to those who are interested. It also sells copies of the privately published *Let Me Die Before I Wake* by Derek Humphry, its president. The book costs $11.50 including postage, and it contains precise instructions for a painless death using readily available ingredients.

In some areas copies of death certificates may be available from funeral directors, morgues, treating hospitals, or physicians; where they are not, see appendix J for ordering information.

Burial Benefits

1. LOCAL PROGRAMS

Almost all local governments bury indigents—and especially indigents who are unidentified or for whom no one assumes responsibility. Usually run by the welfare, health, or coroner's office, these programs (except in some of the largest cities) rarely have coherent, clearly stated eligibility rules; decisions to bury a deceased person and/or to finance burials or funerals are often made on an ad hoc, funds-available basis. In some areas, the understanding has emerged that welfare clients' burials are to be publicly funded, particularly where survivors are welfare recipients themselves. In such cases, the welfare office will typically have contracts with one or more area undertakers; such funerals and burials are quite simple and inexpensive but generally allow for religious or other memorial services, a funeral home viewing or reception, and a spartan but dignified burial. Flowers, elaborate caskets, limousines, and even headstones are rarely provided. Of course, in a few areas provisions might be even more minimal: cremation only, or unceremonious trucking of the remains in a cardboard box to bulldozed mass graves in grim, desolate "Potter's Fields." Donation of the remains for scientific use or for transplantation—other often-used recourses for handling indigents' remains—would generally not be suitable for the HIV-infected.

To secure a locally funded funeral (if available) and burial, one must be careful not to allow hospital or local officials to assume that relatives or friends will handle (and thus be responsible for payment of) arrangements. Probably the best way to proceed (given the ad hoc nature of local burial programs) is to inquire: "What arrangements will the city/county make? *I* can't assume responsibility. I'm on welfare (or whatever program) myself, so *they* will have to bury him, but I would like to pay my respects at a funeral or graveside." This approach will take some persistence and diplomacy. In this way, locally funded funerals/burials can be arranged, ideally with sufficient accommodation of the friends' and family's need to memorialize the deceased.

2. MEMORIAL SOCIETIES

Memorial societies are the lineal descendants of the self-help, friends-and-neighbors home burials of frontier-era America. They are non-profit volunteer associations of members, who, by banding together, are able to make bulk purchases of economical but dignified funeral/burial services from regular community providers for their members. They require a small initial membership fee, and one must pay the eventual (but significantly discounted) funeral costs. To locate a memorial society in your area, contact the Continental Association of Funeral and Memorial Societies, 2001 S Street, N.W., Washington, DC 20009, telephone (202) 462–8888.

3. FUNERAL HOME, UNDERTAKER, AND CEMETERY LICENSURE AGENCIES

All states have agencies which regulate and license funeral homes, undertakers, morticians and cemeteries. Further information about inexpensive arrangements may be available from them; in any case, they handle complaints about sales tactics, prices, quality of arrangements, and grave maintenance. Names and addresses of these boards can be secured through city or county health departments, as well as from local funeral homes.

4. SOCIAL SECURITY ADMINISTRATION (SSA)

The Social Security Administration pays a death or "burial" benefit (currently $255), for a deceased insured person who received or could have received Social Security (but *not* to those who received only SSI), to his or her spouse or children, *but only if the children, too, had been receiving payments on the deceased's record.*

5. DEPARTMENT OF VETERANS AFFAIRS (VA)

The VA provides free burials and gravesites to any veteran, veteran's spouse or widow(er), or minor child at several dozen national cemeteries across the country. Burials are done on a space-available basis; gravesites are no longer available at Arlington National Cemetery (except for high officials and highly decorated veterans) and in much of California. However, niches for cremated remains are available everywhere. Free VA markers and headstones for veterans *are* provided, and these can include not only a name and life dates, but also certain military decorations. The VA pays for transportation to a gravesite of the remains of *those who died in VA hospitals.*

The VA pays $76 (in 1989) toward a nongovernment headstone; it pays $150 for a plot in a nongovernment cemetery for burial of service-connected disability compensation recipients, "wartime" veterans, or indeed any veteran entitled to a burial allowance; it pays $300 for burial to survivors of disability payment recipients, or survivors of *any veteran dying in a VA hospital.* The VA also drapes a deceased veteran's casket with an American flag and arranges for a military honor guard and presentation of the flag to the next of kin or a friend. Finally, the VA will secure a written statement of thanks for the veteran's service, signed by the president on behalf of the nation, for the next of kin or a friend. It is important to note that deceased spouses and children are eligible solely for burial and a gravesite—the other benefits are only for veterans.

Survivor Benefits

Spouses or ex-spouses caring for the minor (or disabled-in-childhood but now grown) children of any covered worker—whether or not he or she actually had a chance to receive SSDI benefits—are eligible for Social Security Survivors Insurance Payments. Eligible also are widows and widowers over 60 and disabled widows, widowers, and divorced spouses over 50 (if unable to claim on their own records). Minors under age 22, or 19 if in school, and adult children with disabilities dating from before age 22 also receive survivors' benefits on a deceased parent's record. It should be noted, too, that any SSDI (but not SSI) check the deceased, insured person received in the month of death must be refunded by the survivors to SSA.

The VA makes survivor payments to spouses and minor or disabled children of veterans who die of a service-connected disability; the amount is determined by the veteran's military pay grade. These benefits are not taxable. Disabled, "wartime-service" pensioners' survivors are also entitled to pensions, if their incomes fall below applicable levels. Moreover, both classes of survivors may be eligible for CHAMPVA, CHAMPUS, or even for military installation health care if space is available (see subsection below).

Spouses, children, and other survivors of deceased PWAs should also be sure to check with former employers and unions to inquire about any death benefits, pensions, or health insurance available from these sources—even if the PWA him or herself received no coverage. Finally, home mortgage, auto loan, and personal loan lenders should be questioned about the possibility of loan payoffs through any credit life insurance they purchased on the deceased.

Taxes

1. MEDICARE INCOME-RELATED PREMIUM

A disabled SSDI recipient who becomes eligible for Medicare was to have paid a surcharge on his or her regular federal income tax beginning with the first *full* year of Medicare eligibility (even if he or she rejects coverage) under the now-repealed Medicare Catastrophic Coverage Act. The additional amount was to have been $22.50 (in 1989) per $150 of regular federal income tax liability, rising to $42 per $150 by 1993. In late 1989, Congress repealed the supplemental Medicare premium tax because of vociferous opposition by affluent elderly persons. It does not even apply for 1989 taxes.

2. PARTIAL TAXATION OF SSDI BENEFIT INCOME

Generally, SSDI benefits are not subject to federal income taxes. However, several years ago the law was amended to tax up to half the SSDI benefits of those who have *otherwise taxable income* of more than $25,000 ($32,000 for a couple). The portion of SSDI benefits subject to the tax rises on a sliding scale. The Internal Revenue Service (IRS) has estimated, however, that only a tiny minority of Social Security recipients will be subject to this provision.

3. HELP WITH TAXES

The IRS operates a Volunteer Income Tax Assistance (VITA) program for disabled persons, which offers free help in preparing federal income tax returns. Call the IRS number listed in the government section of the telephone book, or call (800) 424–1040 for details and arrangements.

4. DISABILITY INCOME TAX CREDIT

Not only does the IRS permit the deduction of most unreimbursed medical expenses in figuring federal income tax liability, but it also provides an income tax credit against tax liability to the permanently and totally disabled. You can order Schedule R, "Credit for the Elderly or Disabled"—which must be countersigned by a doctor certifying the disability—and its instructions, as well as Form 1040 (you can't use the short forms for this) and *its* instructions either from local IRS offices or by calling (800) 424–3676.

5. EARNED INCOME TAX CREDIT FOR THOSE WITH CHILDREN

The earned income tax credit applies to any taxpayer with low or moderate income who (1) had work earnings *for at least part of the year* and (2) was raising one or more children under 18. The credit can be taken by those who cease working for any reason, even to go on SSDI, SSI, or welfare. This provision can not only generate a refund of part or all taxes withheld from paychecks, but *it can generate a "refund" far and above the withheld tax amounts.* In this way, it effectively functions as a "negative income tax," and it can provide real windfalls to needy PWAs and their families. Remember, *any* work earnings during the year (plus having a child) make a taxpayer eligible (if income is otherwise modest). Moreover, earned income tax credit refunds are rarely counted by the SSI, AFDC, Medicaid, and Food Stamp programs. The credit can be computed on the basic 1040, 1040A, and 1040EZ tax forms, which include instructions. For tax year 1988, one's income must have been below $18,576 for one to take the credit, but in late 1989 Congress was moving to liberalize significantly the income threshold.

6. STATE INCOME TAXES
Almost all state income tax systems allow for an exemption or credit to the disabled in computing liability. As with the federal program, a doctor may have to sign the return certifying the disability and supplementary schedules may have to be completed. *Some* states also provide for a state income tax counterpart to the federal earned income credit for workers with children, as well. Contact the local office of the state tax department for details and forms.

7. HOME PROPERTY TAX REDUCTIONS FOR THE DISABLED
A number of states and localities reduce home property taxes for disabled (as well as elderly) persons. Details about the existence of these provisions, and about procedures to utilize them (such as submission of a doctor's statement), are available from city and county real estate tax departments.

Free Legal Services

In 1989 the federal Legal Services Corporation (LSC) funded the operation of about 175 neighborhood legal services offices throughout the country, as well as 15 issue-specific poverty law "think tanks." Neighborhood legal services offices go by a variety of titles but can always be located through the local bar association. They provide free or reduced-fee legal help to low-income people—*especially* in the benefit eligibility areas discussed in this book; they know more about welfare, VA, SSDI, SSI, Medicaid, Food Stamps, and other entitlement programs' eligibility rules and procedures than almost anyone in the community. They are particularly experienced and adept in handling SSDI, SSI, welfare, and Medicaid reconsiderations, hearings, and appeals, and *they should always be consulted when Social Security denies a disability claim.* Moreover, legal services offices have extensive libraries of entitlement advocacy materials, especially National Clearinghouse for Legal Services publications listed in this book's bibliography. Under federal law, LSC-funded programs cannot handle criminal or gay-rights issues, but they *can* represent PWAs in disability discrimination matters.

Legal Aid Societies are privately funded counterparts to neighborhood legal services, and they handle a similar, "welfare-type" caseload with similar expertise. These agencies exist in major cities, but they are less prevalent in rural areas. Because they usually rely on nongovernment charity funding, their capabilities are sometimes less than those of LSC-financed programs. Their names, too, vary considerably, but they can always be located through the local bar association.

Almost all law schools operate legal aid clinics for low-income clients, using the services of second- and third-year students working under the supervision of law professors skilled in poverty law. Unlike LSC programs, law schools determine their own practice, and thus these students can handle criminal and gay-rights issues if they wish. Nonetheless, they tend to specialize in "welfare" law, as well as landlord-tenant and domestic matters. Their expertise about the welfare system does vary, given that the advisers *are* law students rather than full-fledged, specialized lawyers.

In many areas, local bar associations offer referrals to lawyers who provide the poor with free or low-fee representation. Unfortunately, attorneys participating in these programs tend to be general, business, or criminal lawyers with little or no specialized "welfare law" training. In fact, if you've read this far, you probably know far more about entitlement eligibility than most bar association-referred lawyers. Still, for other, general law issues, needy PWAs may wish to utilize these attorneys' services, where available.

Almost everyone receiving, or applying for, SSDI, SSI, welfare, Medicaid, Food Stamps, or VA benefits will generally be eligible for free or very low-fee services from these legal programs; if asked, PWAs should provide verification of income or assets.

Finally, those facing criminal charges can, if needy, receive free legal representation from either a public defender service, or, in areas without such programs, from a court-appointed lawyer. Court staff, police, and bar associations will be familiar with these arrangements.

Special Medical Benefits

CHAMPUS, CHAMPVA, AND SPACE-AVAILABLE CARE
AT MILITARY HOSPITALS

CHAMPUS is a health insurance program established by the federal government, and it provides a coverage package similar to that of Medicare to spouses and minor children of active servicemen, to spouses and children of retired servicemen, and to retired servicemen (including disability retirees). The insurance is free and has no waiting period or preexisting condition limitations.

Details are available from "health benefits officers" at most military medical facilities.

CHAMPVA is a health plan similar to CHAMPUS which the VA offers to spouses and minor children of veterans who receive service-connected disability compensation or disability pensions, or who did so before death. Not all disabled veterans' dependents or survivors are eligible; details about eligibility are available from the VA.

Free, space-available care at military medical facilities is offered when possible to spouses and minor children of active duty soldiers, sailors, and airmen, and also to *retired* servicemen and their dependents. Because it is only offered when space is available, care is not guaranteed in many (if not most) areas; when it is available, it can be sporadic. Dependents and retirees should check with military medical facilities in their area.

BUREAU OF INDIAN AFFAIRS (BIA) AND INDIAN HEALTH SERVICE (IHS)

The federal government funds and operates little-known welfare and health care systems for American Indians and Alaskan Natives who are members of government-recognized tribes or *who are eligible for membership in such tribes*. Tribes determine ancestry requirements and most do not require members to be "full-blooded"—indeed, many have no ancestry minimum, as long as there is *at least one Indian ancestor*. The welfare system functions on and near tribal reservations, is needs-based and operates through federal BIA or tribal offices. The IHS is a program similar to a health maintenance organization, offering medical care at federal or tribal hospitals on or near reservations (emergency and specialized care is purchased by the IHS from other hospitals in many cases). The IHS, unlike most health plans, provides outpatient prescription drugs, dental care, eyeglasses, and drug/alcohol treatment. Members of American Indian tribes, *as well as those eligible for membership in a tribe*, can receive free health care; this is *not* a needs-based program.

Those with at least one Indian ancestor can call the BIA at (202) 343–1710 for assistance in contacting the office of the tribe for which they may have membership eligibility. To find out about locations of IHS facilities, call (301) 443–1116 (the IHS *does* have several clinics in large cities, and hospitals are within easy commuting distance of metropolitan areas in the Upper Great Lakes, the Mountain states, and the West Coast).

EXTRA HEALTH SERVICES FOR MEDICARE PATIENTS is available where the Health Care Financing Administration (HCFA) contracts with health maintenance organizations (HMOs) for the enrollment of Medicare recipients. For a small additional cost, or sometimes for no fee at all, Medicare enrollees in HMOs not only are relieved from paying deductibles and coinsurance, but they also get free or very low cost outpatient prescriptions, dental care, eyeglasses, and other items that may be included in the HMO package—items currently unavailable to regular Medicare eligibles. Those interested in HMO enrollment should contact their local Social Security office or call (800) 234–5772 for further information. In some areas, comparable arrangements are made for Medicaid recipients, too—check with the welfare office.

FREE DENTAL CARE
Most Medicaid programs do not cover adult dental care, and neither do Medicare or most private health insurance plans. However, free or reduced-price dental treatment is almost always offered by dental schools, which need patients on whom their students may "practice" (under close supervision of dentist-instructors). Waiting lists are long for these programs, and treatments take a very long time, as students must be checked upon by instructors at each step. In addition, free care from participating dentists can be arranged for needy disabled patients through the National Foundation of Dentistry for the Handicapped, 1600 Stout Street, Denver, CO 80202, telephone (303) 573–0264. This program now covers only about 10 states, but it is slowly growing.

MEDIC ALERT IDENTIFICATION necklaces and bracelets for chronically ill people are particularly useful in providing quick information to emergency caregivers. They are available for $25 from the Medic Alert Foundation, P.O. Box 1009, Turlock, CA 96381, telephone (800) 344–3226, in California, (800) 468–1020.

EYEGLASSES, at no cost to the patient, can be arranged for by many local Lions Clubs, which traditionally purchase eyeglasses and related care for the needy. Lions Clubs International, 300 22nd Street, Oak Brook, IL 60570, telephone (312) 986–1730, can provide leads to Lion's Clubs active in your area.

BLIND AND VISION-IMPAIRED PWAs (for example, afflicted by cytomegalovirus retinitis) can receive free referral to specialized social work, mobility and self-care training, and related services through the American Council of the Blind, 1010 Vermont Avenue, N.W., Washington, DC 20005, telephone (202) 393–3666 or (800) 424–8666. Referrals for seeing-eye dog placements are made by the Guide Dog Foundation for the Blind, 171 East Jericho Turnpike, Smithtown, NY 11787, telephone (516) 265–2121. Finally, Canine Companions for Independence, P.O. Box 446, Santa Rosa, CA 95402, telephone (707)

528–0830, provides guide dogs to all types of handicapped persons—not just to the blind.

Special Disability Benefits

BUS AND SUBWAY FARE DISCOUNTS TO THE DISABLED (50%) are offered by almost all local mass transit systems (those with federal funding are required to do so by the U.S. Department of Transportation). In some areas, disabled applicants can present letters from the VA, SSDI, SSI, AFDC, Medicaid, or GA which award benefits on the basis of disability or incapacity. In other areas, a copy of the doctor's report which secured public benefits in the first place must be presented. Finally, some local agencies insist on having their own disability form completed by an applicant's doctor. Call the local transit authority to find out which application procedure is employed in your area. Those found eligible are given handicapped identification cards entitling them to purchase discount tokens and fare cards at transit offices and some banks.

TRAVEL ASSISTANCE is offered by Amtrak, which has discounts of approximately 25% for disabled persons presenting disability award letters from public benefit programs (not available on already discounted excursions). Airlines almost always provide free inter-terminal transport, wheelchairs, and even oxygen; fare discounts vary enormously from airline to airline (check with a travel agent). Several recent law cases have compelled airlines to extend "frequent flyer" bonus flight offerings to gay couples on the same basis as heterosexual families. While Greyhound and Trailways bus lines do not offer fare discounts to the disabled, they do provide a second, *free* fare where a disabled traveler presents a doctor's statement that he is disabled and must have a travel companion. National Parks and other federal recreation and wilderness lands admit disabled people (and those entering in the same vehicle with them) at no charge if they present a disability award letter from any federal program.

VOTING REGISTRATION, at home or by mail, is available in most states, and all states will arrange for absentee voting by the disabled. Telephone the local voting registrar's office, or the League of Women Voters, to make arrangements well before election day.

For advice about issues one might bear in mind while voting, turn to the following chapter.

Improving the System in Your State

Those who have read this far will likely be confused by the dizzying variations in benefit programs from state to state, particularly in the complex interrelationships between SSI, Medicaid, and the state welfare systems. The range of state policy choices means that almost all states have made bad decisions— from the point of view of PWAs—on a variety of issues.

There are improvements that can be made in the way SSI, State Supplements, Medicaid, and welfare work to bring better income and medical care to PWAs—and, indeed, to *all* the needy disabled and elderly people in your state. Some of these changes will cost money, but many of them will be cost-neutral *or even save money*. They need to be brought to the attention of state welfare and Medicaid policy makers, state legislative health and welfare committees, state legislators, and potential allies in senior citizens', disability, mental health/retardation, and health advocacy organizations (see appendix G–2).

Where information and technical assistance can be secured from the federal Department of Health and Human Services (HHS) for SSI, State Supplementary Payment (SSP), or Medicaid issues, appendix F provides the addresses and telephone numbers of the HHS regional offices serving the various states. Raising these issues in both the state health/welfare and the HHS bureaucracies will likely require some persistence, especially to locate the particular individual responsible for each eligibility option or issue; often only a specialist—and not simply a program generalist—will even *understand* the issue, much less have policy responsibility for it.

What follows is a list of the most important income and medical care issues that need improvement or changes. Each issue or proposed change is numbered; the numbers are used to indicate the states in which each change is needed, in the table that follows.

1. **Urge your state to amend its medical licensure statutes to require—as a condition of new or renewed licensure—that *all* medical practitioners and institutions in the state participate in Medicare and Medicaid, and that they accept Medicare and Medicaid fee schedules.**
   Medicare fee schedules, because of the law's computation methodology and

federal funding shortages, *are significantly below what private health insurance and cash patients pay.* As a result, many doctors and other practitioners—in some areas most—refuse to accept Medicare assignment (and thus its fee limits). Moreover, even where a patient has a private health policy in addition to Medicare, the "fine print" terms of such policies adopt the Medicare fees for dual enrollees—even though higher fees are otherwise payable under policies. Thus, even a previously privately insured patient who becomes a Medicare-eligible will suffer from discrimination against low-paying Medicare patients.

For Medicaid patients, the situation, if anything, is even worse: federal law limits Medicaid fees to the Medicare schedule (and many states pay *even less*), thus subjecting Medicaid patients to a low-fee discrimination even more intense than that against Medicare patients; federal law already requires that providers accept Medicaid fees as payments in full; and, in addition, Medicaid patients suffer from traditional prejudice against "welfare" and minority groups. Finally, it should be added that some nursing homes, hospices, home health agencies, pharmacies, and even a few hospitals refuse to participate in Medicare and/or Medicaid.

All of this creates some severe access-to-care problems for PWAs as well as for other needy and disabled persons. Of course, this reluctance of many medical providers raises basic questions about adherence to the Hippocratic Oath and about recent health care expansion programs endorsed by organized medicine. Several New England states have moved to resolve these access problems by requiring, as a condition of licensure, the acceptance of Medicare assignment; there have also been moves similarly to mandate acceptance of Medicaid patients. See note 2 in Medicare section.

Contact the Villers Foundation for *The Best Medicine* ($7.50), a health access promotion manual; the American Medical Association for the free *Health Policy Agenda* materials; and the National Clearinghouse for Legal Services for *Doctors for the Poor: Increasing Physician Participation in Medicaid* ($10.50; order no. 43,205).

Lobby state health licensure and Medicaid officials, state health legislative committees, and members of the legislature. Seek allies in public health, hospital, doctors', religious, senior citizens', disability, and mental health/retardation advocacy groups.

2. Urge your state Medicaid program to secure a "Section 2176" waiver from HHS to offer "home and community-based services" to PWAs and other disabled people as an alternative to more expensive and more personally disruptive hospitalization or nursing home placement.

This kind of program will improve the quality of life for PWAs and other disabled and aged people—and it will save the state money it now spends on hospital and nursing home bills. This will enable the state to offer far more home health, personal care attendant, chore aid, homemaker, and other supportive services than are ordinarily covered in its Medicaid package. It could also permit some broadening of eligibility, as well. Contact the National AIDS Network for a "how-to" manual on *2176 Waivers* ($15.00), and the Villers Foundation for *The Best Medicine* ($7.50), a waiver-promotion manual.

Lobby state Medicaid officials, state health and welfare legislative committees, and members of the legislature. Seek allies in senior citizens', disability, religious, and mental health/retardation advocacy groups. Contact your regional HHS office.

3. **Urge your state Medicaid program to add coverage of the "medically needy"—these are disabled people who are "too rich" for SSI or welfare, but still poor enough to need medical help. The federal government offers to help all states cover these people, but your state has so far not acted to cover them.**

Currently, in your state, those with income above the SSI or welfare level are "too rich" for Medicaid—even if their incomes are only $1 over the SSI level. If the state took the "medically needy" option, such persons could "spend down" to become poor enough for Medicaid, even if they start out with incomes which are "too high" (see Medicaid section). While this proposal would cost more state money, it would also save money: the medical care of presently uncovered "medically needy" people is *already included* in the charity budgets of city, county, state, state university, and other publicly subsidized hospitals. And the state may already be paying some of these costs through higher hospital billings to Medicaid (because of the many uncollectible debts hospitals absorb and pass on from people who could be covered as "medically needy"). There's also something unjust in giving Medicaid only to those "on welfare" while denying it to those who worked hard enough to generate an income above the welfare level.

Contact the Villers Foundation for *The Best Medicine,* a "medically needy" program promotion manual, the American Hospital Association for *Medicaid Options: Expanding Eligibility* (free), the American Medical Association for the free *Health Policy Agenda* materials on Medicaid reform, and the National Clearinghouse for Legal Services for *Adopting a Medically Needy Program* (Dec. 1984); $6.00.

Lobby state Medicaid officials, state health and welfare legislative committees, and members of the legislature. Seek allies in hospital, public health, doctors', religious, senior citizens', disability, and mental health/retardation advocacy groups. Contact regional HHS office.

4. **Urge your state to sign agreements with the Social Security Administration under Sections 1616 and 1634 of the Social Security Act for simultaneous, automatic determinations of SSI, SSP, and Medicaid eligibility. The federal government would pay most or all of the administrative costs (see SSP and Medicaid sections, and appendix B-1.)**

In *most* states, the SSI eligibility determination simultaneously constitutes an SSP and Medicaid eligibility determination. SSA sends lists of new and continuing SSI and SSP eligibles to the state and the state automatically mails Medicaid cards to them (under Section 1634) and reimburses SSA for the SSP money paid to them (under Section 1616). This means that PWAs and other disabled people do simple, "one-stop shopping," and they don't have to go through the ordeal of two separate eligibility applications at two separate offices.

Your state rejected these "1616" and "1634" options; it is either a "209(b)" state (using eligibility rules slightly stricter than SSI's in a few unimportant ways) or a "Title XVI" state (accepting SSI rules, but still requiring that SSI applicants apply separately for Medicaid at the welfare office). Or, even if it is a "1634" state, some or all of its SSPs have to be applied for separately at the welfare office. This means that each and every month, thousands of PWAs and other needy disabled and aged people are shuttling back and forth between SSA and welfare offices; a blizzard of verification forms, notes, and telephone calls passes unnecessarily between these offices to inquire about and verify an applicant's status; hundreds of welfare waiting rooms are cluttered up with disabled and aged people filing "duplicate" applications; and uncounted thousands of hours of welfare workers' time is consumed by this "artificial" caseload.

The eligibility change to full "1616" and "1634" status will cost the state little or nothing (your state's Medicaid and SSP rules are *already* identical, or nearly identical, to SSI's anyway). But the change will *save money and welfare employees' time* by eliminating unnecessary duplicate applications, liaisons, and paperwork. In addition, it is simply indefensible to require the sickest, most infirm people in the state to run the already intolerable eligibility determination gauntlet *twice*. This change will free up scarce, overworked, and underpaid welfare workers for more meaningful, productive work.

Lobby state Medicaid and welfare officials, state health and welfare legislative committees, and members of the legislature. Seek allies in religious, senior citizens', disability, and mental health/retardation advocacy groups. Contact regional HHS office.

5. **Urge the state to raise to more adequate levels (or begin paying, if not yet doing so) its State Supplementary Payment (SSP) for PWAs and**

other disabled and aged people living in board and care homes (see Board and Care Home section and appendix B–1). Urge streamlining of state licensure rules for board and care homes to permit easier, simpler start-up of group homes for PWAs and other needy disabled people. Seek state help in paying for start-up, equipping, and staffing costs of PWA board and care homes.

Many PWAs and other disabled persons have nowhere to live or, for reasons of infirmity, *must* live in group housing such as board and care homes. States need to pay an adequate SSP on top of the basic federal SSI level, however, to give these residents enough "rent" money to cover the higher living costs in these specially equipped, specially staffed facilities. State licensure requirements need to be simple and streamlined enough to allow board and care homes to begin operation without a lot of bureaucratic red tape or overly technical architectural, staffing, or equipment standards. States need to make grants or loans available for board and care home start-up costs, using funds from housing laws, the federal Homeless Act, or other sources.

How does your state stack up on all these issues? Don't forget that board and care homes (and adequate SSPs for their needy residents to pay "rent") are *realistic alternatives* to costly, more socially disruptive placement in hospitals, nursing homes, and hospices; an effective program gives infirm and/or homeless PWAs a protected, supervised, home-like setting—*and it saves the state substantial medical costs.* Contact the National Association for Residential Care Facilities for information and advice about streamlining board and care home licensure and assistance in your state; the American Association of Retired Persons (AARP) for *A Home Away From Home,* a manual/resource book, for *Preserving Independence, Supporting Needs,* and for *The Board and Care System: A Regulatory Jungle* (all free); the American Bar Association for *An Addendum to the Model Act: Financial Incentives for Board and Care Facilities* (Dec. 1984), a review of ways to finance these facilities; and the Massachusetts Department of Elder Affairs for *Independence Through Interdependence,* a free "how-to" manual on setting up a board and care home.

Lobby state welfare, group home licensure, Medicaid, and housing officials, state health, welfare, and housing legislative committees, and members of the legislature. Seek allies in senior citizens', religious, disability, and mental health/retardation advocacy groups. Contact regional HHS office.

6. Urge your state to establish a general prescription drug assistance program for moderate-income, disabled, and aged people who are "too rich" for Medicaid.

Nine states already have such programs (see AZT/Drug section). But the cost of AZT and other AIDS drugs is a real burden for those PWAs who are "slightly too rich" for Medicaid. This is all the more true now that the specially funded federal AZT assistance program faces phase-out in the annual Congressional appropriations battles. Contact the Villers Foundation for *The Best Medicine,* a drug program advocacy manual.

Lobby state Medicaid, health and welfare officials, state health and welfare legislative committees, and members of the legislature. Seek allies in pharmaceutical firms, pharmacists' associations, drug store chains, senior citizens', religious, disability, and mental health/retardation advocacy groups. Contact state drug programs listed in the AZT/Drug section for information on existing programs.

7. **Urge your state to give full Medicaid coverage to all disabled and aged persons with income below the federal poverty level (about $522 monthly for one person in early 1990, but updated annually by cost of living increase). Federal law already gives states the option of doing this with federal help.**

This change would give Medicaid to many, many more near-needy PWAs and other disabled and aged people, because the federal poverty level is *significantly above* the SSI, SSI/SSP, or Medicaid-only eligibility levels most states now use to decide who gets Medicaid. Moreover, it makes a good deal of administrative sense for states to do this: a new federal law, effective January 1, 1990, requires them to have their Medicaid programs pay *Medicare* premiums, co-payments, and deductibles for aged and disabled Medicare beneficiaries with incomes below 90% of the poverty level (100% of the poverty level by 1992). Thus, state welfare departments are already required to do these special "90% of poverty" Medicaid/Medicare eligibility determinations *anyway;* their welfare workers already are, or shortly will be, burdened with this additional workload.

Why go to the trouble of making Medicaid eligibility determinations for these people, but then using Medicaid money only for *Medicare* premiums, co-payments, and deductibles? Why not cover them for *all* Medicaid services? It won't cost much, since almost all the aged and disabled are already on Medicare and Medicare pays almost all their medical costs now anyway (except for a few "extras"). But these few "extras" (medical costs Medicaid will have to pay because Medicare doesn't cover them *at all,* such as prescription drugs) make a big difference to poor aged and disabled people.

And these costs make an even bigger difference to needy PWAs because many of them—*unlike* almost all the other disabled and the aged—are *not on Medicare yet because of the 2-year waiting period.* Thus, if a state takes this option, it can make all the difference in the world for poor, but currently ineligible, PWAs who would thereby get desperately necessary Medicaid coverage.

Contact the regional HHS office for more information on this complex but vital provision. You can secure a set of advocacy brochures on this provision by requesting free "QMB" packets from the Villers Foundation. Both the National Health Care Campaign and the American Hospital Association have *Medicaid Expansion* manuals on this issue as well.

Lobby state Medicaid officials, state health and welfare legislative committees, and members of the legislature. Seek allies in hospital, doctors', pharmacists', drug merchandisers', religious, senior citizens', disability, and mental health/retardation advocacy groups.

8. **Urge your state to begin paying—or increase existing—State Supplementary Payments (SSPs) for needy disabled and aged people living in their own homes.**

Can a needy PWA or other disabled or aged person really survive on the currently paid SSI ($386 in 1990) or combined SSI/SSP amount in your state? Can anyone realistically even pay rent, much less buy food, furnish a home and wardrobe, or pay for simple entertainment on this amount? It is a disgrace how pitifully low living allowances are for poor disabled and aged people (and they're *even lower* in the AFDC and General Assistance welfare programs!).

States can begin paying—or increase already existing—SSPs to cover realistic living expenses. The Social Security Administration will even do all the administrative and eligibility determination work for the state—and bill it later for the extra SSP monies it pays out. In fact, states (with the agreement of the U.S. Departments of Health and Human Services and Agriculture) can do this at *no* cost to them at all by using existing demonstrations authority in federal laws to finance SSPs—or raise existing SSP levels—by converting the averaged cash value of Food Stamps into SSPs (or *increased* SSPs). In this way, a higher income can be paid, the necessity of a separate Food Stamps application at the welfare office for SSI recipients can be obviated, and the resultant, higher combined SSI/SSP level—derived wholly from "cashed-out," federally financed Food Stamp funds—can even thereby serve as a new and more generous Medicaid income level.

Here is an example. The combined SSI/SSP/Medicaid level in 1990 in the District of Columbia is $401, as D.C. has already taken the "1616" and "1634" options for SSA to administer eligibility for its SSPs and Medicaid. The estimated maximum value of Food Stamps for an SSI/SSP recipient in D.C. with higher than average shelter costs is $61 (see appendix B–2), which we will assume for the sake of argument will become the "averaged out" Food

Stamp allotment of typical SSI/SSP residents in D.C. The city could secure federal approval for a demonstration to add the $61 value to the combined SSI/SSP standard of $401, for a new total level of $462, with the additional SSP amount actually derived from Food Stamp funds. And, as D.C. is a "1634" state, the new combined SSI/(enhanced) SSP level also serves as the Medicaid level. Moreover, applicants would no longer have to visit the welfare office separately.

While the increased regular SSPs will mean more welfare expenses for the state budget, the more stable and healthy living conditions thereby promoted will *save* state Medicaid, institutional, shelter, and emergency assistance costs now being paid out. Moreover, the state could limit the impact of a new (or increased) SSP on the welfare budget by making it payable only to those living on their own in higher-cost housing (that is, now-poor PWAs living in middle-income apartments or homes they secured before they stopped working due to illness).

Lobby state Medicaid and welfare officials, state health and welfare legislative committees, and members of the legislature. Seek allies in senior citizens', religious, disability, and mental health/retardation advocacy groups. Contact the regional HHS office.

9. Urge your state to begin paying—or to raise to adequate levels—a statewide, uniform-across-county-lines General Assistance (GA) welfare grant to needy, incapacitated persons who are not quite "disabled enough" for SSI, or who are waiting for delayed SSI eligibility determinations (see General Assistance and SSI sections).

Some states have no General Assistance (GA) grants at all for the needy "near-disabled" or those whose applications are pending with SSI. Others have inadequate GA grants, or GA grants payable only at *county* option, or GA programs with unusually burdensome eligibility rules (such as forbidding home or car ownership or small "nest eggs"). Many PWAs "pending" with SSI—plus *most* "ARC-only" patients—have to depend on state GA programs for minimal living expenses. Where GA grants are nonexistent or too low, not available in *all* counties, or burdened with excessive eligibility limits, needy "PWAs-pending-with-SSI" and PWARCs—as well as other needy disabled and aged people in similar situations—have serious problems in meeting living expenses.

A good case can be made to improve—or to create for the first time—a state GA program because we're talking here not about "welfare," or "welfare mothers" (unpopular topics nowadays), but about minimal "disability payments" to those medically unable to work. (True, state GA disability standards are *more liberal* than those of SSI, but they still usually involve *some* determination about medical inability to work.) Also, this GA issue can be "sold" to states because of the (supposedly effective) arrangement state welfare departments can make to get back the GA money they "advance" to "SSI-pending" applicants whose applications SSI finally approves (see General Assistance and SSI sections).

Lobby state welfare officials, state welfare legislative committees, and members of the legislature. Seek allies in senior citizens', religious, disability, and mental health/retardation advocacy groups.

10. **Urge your state to adopt a new—or improve an inadequate—General Medical Assistance/Indigent Medical Care program for poor people who are not the *kinds* of people (disabled under SSDI/SSI definition) covered by federal Medicaid—and to offer benefits similar to Medicaid in this state program.**

Some states have no real medical assistance program similar to Medicaid to cover poor people not covered by Medicaid; such persons must seek free or inexpensive care—often on an emergency-admission basis—as charity cases at city, county, state, state university, or (where accessible) private hospitals and clinics. Other states make such medical assistance for these people optional by county; thus it is unavailable in conservative or poor counties. Still others offer a watered down medical assistance program, with services limited to public hospitals and clinics; or these people may only get care as authorized on a "treatment-by-treatment" or "funds-available" basis. Many programs have serious coverage gaps (such as covering only inpatient hospital care, or not covering prescriptions at all). In addition, some make *no* provision for covering persons with incomes above the welfare level through a "spend down" provision like that of Medicaid.

And, finally, some states have so-called "indigent care" programs, for poor, non-Medicaid-type people, which only subsidize hospital "bad debt" losses,[1] but which make no meaningful provision for continuing, routine, non-emergency access to care (such as giving people Medicaid-type cards with which to purchase routine as well as emergency care). In fact, the so-called "bad debt/charity care" for which hospitals get public subsidies or rate allowances under these schemes *do not* even stipulate that the "bad debt/charity care" an indigent patient receives is to be canceled as a debt without referral to a collection agency or credit bureau. Unfortunately, this particular way of establishing

---

1. These are losses due to debts run up where hospitals are forced to admit, on an emergency basis, poor people with no coverage who are later (naturally) unable to pay their bills.

or expanding state indigent care programs is now currently in vogue in most states—even though it is the least beneficial to indigent people on the issues of continuing access to care, credit ratings, and debt collection.

The problem is that many PWAs and PWARCs—unlike the *traditional* poor (who have *no* assets and whose pitifully low, irregular salaries are not worth garnishing)—may have equity in homes, or small liquid assets which "bad debt" in credit files *will* endanger. Since many currently fashionable "indigent care" programs (1) don't guarantee continuing access to ongoing routine care (as federal Medicaid does) and (2) endanger the small home equities and assets some PWAs hope to leave to loved ones, states need to replace or expand them with something similar to *federal* Medicaid.

This *will* be a very expensive proposition; on the other hand, public opinion is now more receptive to doing something meaningful about this problem than it has been in years.

Lobby state Medicaid, health, welfare, and insurance officials; state health, welfare, and insurance legislative committees; and members of the legislature. Seek allies in health insurance, hospital, physicians', senior citizens', religious, disability, and mental health/retardation advocacy groups. Contact the National Health Care Campaign for the *Insuring the Uninsured: Options for State Action* manual ($25.00) and the American Medical Association for the free *Health Policy Agenda* materials package. Secure technical advice from state Medicaid officials in states which already operate "Medicaid-like" programs to cover their non-federal-type poor people: New York, Maryland, and California already have good programs for these people.

Necessary Improvements, State-by-State

State	Improvements (described in chapter)									
	1	2	3	4	5	6	7	8	9	10
AL	•	•	•		•	•	•	•	•	•
AK	•	•	•	•	•	•				
AZ	•	•			•	•	•	•		
AR	•	•			•	•	•	•	•	•
CA	•				•	•				
CO	•	•	•	•	•	•	•	•		•
CT	•	•		•	•		•			
DE	•	•	•		•		•	•	•	•
DC	•	•			•	•		•		
FL	•				•	•		•	•	•
GA	•	•	•		•	•	•	•	•	•

State	Improvements (described in chapter)									
	1	2	3	4	5	6	7	8	9	10
HI	•			•²	•	•	•	•		
ID	•	•	•	•	•	•	•	•	•	•
IL	•			•	•		•	•		
IN	•	•	•³	•	•	•	•	•	•	•
IA	•	•			•	•	•	•	•	•
KS	•	•		•²	•	•	•	•	•	
KY	•	•			•	•	•	•	•	•
LA	•	•			•	•	•	•	•	•
ME	•	•			•		•	•	•	
MD	•	•			•		•	•	•	
MA	•	•			•	•	•			
MI	•	•			•	•	•	•		
MN	•	•		•	•	•	•	•		
MS	•	•	•		•	•	•	•	•	•
MO	•	•	•³	•	•	•	•	•	•	
MT	•	•			•	•	•	•	•	
NE	•	•		•	•	•	•	•	•	
NV	•	•	•	•²	•	•	•	•	•	•
NH	•	•		•	•	•	•	•	•	•
NJ	•				•			•		
NM	•		•		•	•	•	•	•	•
NY	•	•			•		•			
NC	•			•	•	•	•	•	•	•
ND	•	•		•	•	•	•	•	•	•
OH	•		•³	•	•	•	•	•		

2. State *does* have "1616" contract with SSA for simultaneous SSI/SSP determinations at SSA office, but does *not* have "1634" contract with SSA for simultaneous SSI/Medicaid eligibility determinations; hence, all disabled and aged applicants must also visit welfare office to apply for Medicaid.

3. These states do *not* now have "medically needy" programs, even though they *do* have "spend down" eligibility for aged and disabled people with incomes over the state Medicaid level. However, their current "spend downs" are legally required of them as "209(b)" states (states having *some* eligibility rule(s) stricter than those of SSI). Since issue #4 calls for these states to end their "209(b)" status by becoming "1634" states (giving Medicaid automatically to all SSI recipients), it follows that they will have to take the "medically needy" option to preserve the "spend down" method of becoming eligible for those aged and disabled persons with income over the Medicaid level.

State	Improvements (described in chapter)									
	1	2	3	4	5	6	7	8	9	10
OK	●	●		●	●	●	●	●	●	●
OR	●	●		●	●	●	●	●		
PA	●				●					
RI	●	●			●					
SC	●		●		●	●	●	●	●	●
SD	●	●	●	●[4]	●	●	●	●	●	●
TN	●	●			●	●	●	●	●	●
TX	●	●	●		●	●	●	●	●	●
UT	●	●		●	●	●	●	●	●	●
VT	●	●			●	●	●			
VA	●	●		●	●	●	●	●	●	●
WA	●	●			●	●	●	●		
WV	●	●			●	●	●	●	●	●
WI	●	●			●	●	●			
WY	●	●	●	●	●	●	●	●	●	●

Source: Adapted by author from data reported by states to the Social Security Administration (SSA) and the Health Care Financing Administration (HCFA) of the U.S. Department of Health and Human Services (HHS), as of mid-1989.

4. State *does* have "1634" contract with SSA for simultaneous SSI/Medicaid eligibility determinations at SSA office, but does *not* have "1616" contract with SSA for simultaneous SSI/SSP eligibility determinations for its general SSPs; hence, some or all disabled and aged applicants must also visit welfare office to apply for SSPs.

Appendix A

AZT Drug Program Contact Telephone Numbers, by State

Alabama
(205) 261–5016
Alaska
(907) 561–4406
Arizona
(602) 255–1024
Arkansas
(501) 661–2315
California
(916) 445–0553
Colorado
(303) 294–2541
Connecticut
(203) 566–1874
Delaware
(302) 736–5617
District of Columbia
(202) 673–7700
Florida
(904) 487–2478
Georgia
(404) 894–5304
Hawaii
(808) 524–4899
Idaho
(208) 334–5941
Illinois
(217) 785–2955
Indiana
(317) 232–4391
Iowa
(515) 281–4936
(800) 532–3301

Kansas
(913) 296–5585
Kentucky
(502) 564–4478
Louisiana
(504) 568–5005
Maine
(207) 289–3591
(800) 452–1999
(weekend emergencies)
Maryland
(301) 225–6742
Massachusetts
(617) 727–0049
Michigan
(517) 334–7204
Minnesota
(612) 297–3200
Mississippi
(601) 961–7725
Missouri
(314) 751–6146
Montana
(406) 444–4740
Nebraska
(402) 471–2937
Nevada
(702) 885–4730
New Hampshire
(603) 271–4602
New Jersey
(609) 292–5050

New Mexico
(505) 827–4483
New York
(518) 474–8162
(800) 542–2437
North Carolina
(919) 733–3419
North Dakota
(701) 224–2378
Ohio
(614) 466–6420
(from out of state only)
(800) 282–1190 x 6420
(within state only)
Oklahoma
(405) 271–4060
Oregon
(503) 229–5792
Pennsylvania
(717) 787–5900
Puerto Rico
(809) 751–4908
Rhode Island
(401) 277–2362
South Carolina
(803) 734–5020
South Dakota
(605) 773–3357
Tennessee
(615) 741–7247
Texas
(800) 255–1090

Utah	Virgin Islands	Wisconsin
(801) 538–6495	(809) 773–1059	(608) 266–5482
Vermont	Washington	Wyoming
(802) 241–2880	(206) 586–0427	(307) 777–7953
Virginia	West Virginia	
(800) 533–4148	(304) 348–8990	

Source: Adapted by author from listing prepared by the AIDS staff of the Health Resources and Services Administration (HRSA), Public Health Services (PHS), U.S. Department of Health and Human Services (HHS), as of 1988.

Note: When telephoning these numbers, ask where and how to apply in person in your local area, if possible; if it is not, ask how to apply by mail, and to what central address; give your name and address in order to receive mailed application forms; inquire what documentation you need to submit with your application; ask about what drugs other than AZT are covered; find out what the income and asset eligibility rules are; and, finally, ask how the AZT Drug Program may match up with any health insurance you may have.

Appendix B

SSI/SSP and Food Stamp Allotments and Computation

State Supplementary Payments (SSPs) to SSI for 1990, by State

Total Combined SSI and State Supplementary Payment (SSP) Eligibility and Payment Level (in dollars)[1]

State	Living Independently	Living in Board and Care Home[2]
AL	386[3]	442 +
AK	701[4]	701
AZ	386[3]	436
AR	386[3]	386[3]
CA	620	696 +
CO	390[4]	581 +
CT	*[4]	*
DE	386[3]	526
DC	401	533.20 +
FL	386[3]	472 +
GA	386[3]	386 +
HI	390.90	580.90
ID	459[4]	511 +
IL	*[4]	*
IN	386[3]	*
IA	386[3]	448.20 +
KS	386[3]	386[3] +
KY	386[3]	480 +
LA	386[3]	386[3]
ME	396	442 +
MD	386[3]	465.50 +
MA	500.39	557.58 +
MI	416.20	473 +
MN	421[4]	*

State	Living Independently	Living in Board and Care Home[2]
MS	386[3]	386[3]
MO	386[3]	530
MT	386[3]	480
NE	424[4]	390+
NV	386[3]	386[3]
NH	413[4]	554+
NJ	417.25	536.05+
NM	386[3]	461
NY	452[5]	634.96+
NC	386[3]	705+
ND	386[3]	*
OH	386[3]	496+
OK	450[4]	450+
OR	387.70[4]	387.70+
PA	418.40	533.30
RI	444.55	444.55+
SC	386[3]	*
SD	386[5]	*
TN	386[3]	386[3]
TX	386[3]	386[3]
UT	394.80	394.80+
VT	446.10	480.20+
VA	386[3]	468+
WA	414	414+
WV	386[3]	703+
WI	488.72	589.16+
WY	406[4]	406[4]

Source: Adapted and estimated (by adding 1989 SSP dollar amounts to the 1990 basic federal SSI level) by author from data reported by states, through late 1989, to Social Security Administration (SSA), U.S. Department of Health and Human Services (HHS), updated through conversations with staff of the HHS's Health Care Financing Administration (HCFA), and augmented by author's personal files.

[1] The combined SSI and SSP amount is also the Medicaid income level here.

[2] In all states, board and care home residents apply for the SSP at the local welfare office.

[3] SSI amount only; no SSP is paid.

[4] In these states, apply to SSA for SSI amount, but to local welfare office for SSP amount.

[5] In addition to the federally administered SSI/SSP level shown here, New York City pays an additional *city* SSP—to PWAs only—through its welfare offices, for a combined, total SSI/SSP/"city" SSP benefit level of about $760. South Dakota also pays a $15 SSP to disabled persons living independently, but only if they qualify for the basic federal SSI to begin with.

+ Even higher SSP can sometimes be paid to those in more supportive or larger board and care homes.

* SSP above the SSI level is paid, but there is no set, statewide SSP level; instead, an individually tailored SSP level is applied to each applicant.

Note: No SSI/SSP levels are shown for Guam, Puerto Rico, and the Virgin Islands, because different (and far lower) income programs for the poor disabled operate there.

Maximum Possible Food Stamp Allotments for Single SSI/SSP Recipients, 1989, by State (in dollars)

AL	66	KY	66	ND	66
AK	55[1,3]	LA	66	OH	66
AZ	66	ME	63	OK	46
AR	66	MD	66	OR	65
CA	0[2]	MA	27	PA	56
CO	48	MI	57	RI	47
CT	na[3]	MN	na[3]	SC	66
DE	66	MS	66	SD	61
DC	61	MO	66	TN	66
FL	66	MT	66	TX	66
GA	66	NE	54	UT	63
HI	137[1]	NV	66	VT	48
ID	50	NH	61	VA	66
IL	na[3]	NJ	56	WA	57
IN	66	NM	66	WV	66
IA	66	NY	40	WI	0[2]
KS	66	NC	66	WY	60

Source: Adapted by author from U.S. House of Representatives, Committee on Ways and Means, *Background Material and Data on Programs Within the Jurisdiction of the Committe on Ways and Means,* March 15, 1989, 681–82.

[1] Food Stamp allocations are higher in Alaska and Hawaii than in the continental states. But this table does not show the higher maximum possible allotments because the higher the SSP (or *any* income), the more it depresses the Food Stamp allotment.

[2] SSI/SSP recipients in California and Wisconsin get bigger cash SSP benefits in lieu of Food Stamps.

[3] Because the state-administered SSPs in these states can in many cases be raised to accommodate higher shelter costs, resultant Food Stamp allocations are unpredictable; those receiving fairly generous SSPs to meet shelter costs could, in some cases, thereby have their Food Stamp allocation reduced to zero.

Note: Puerto Rico has a different food assistance program.

Food Stamp Program: Monthly Allotments and Deductions, October 1989–September 1990

Maximum Food Stamp Allotments (in dollars)

Household Size	48 States and DC	Alaska	Hawaii	Guam	Virgin Islands
1	99	123	151	146	127
2	182	227	276	268	234
3	260	325	396	384	335
4	331	413	503	488	425
5	393	490	598	579	505
6	472	588	717	695	606
7	521	650	793	768	670
8	596	743	906	878	766
Each additional member	+75	+93	+113	+110	+96

Deductions (in dollars)

Area	Standard Deductions
48 States and DC	112
Alaska	191
Hawaii	158
Guam	224
Virgin Islands	98

Net Monthly Income Eligibility Standards (100% of Poverty Level, in dollars)

Household Size	48 States[1]	Alaska	Hawaii
1	499	624	573
2	669	836	769
3	839	1,049	965
4	1,009	1,261	1,160
5	1,179	1,474	1,356
6	1,349	1,686	1,552
7	1,519	1,899	1,748
8	1,689	2,111	1,944
Each additional member	+170	+213	+196

Source: Food and Nutrition Service, U.S. Department of Agriculture.
[1] Same levels prevail in District of Columbia, Guam, and the Virgin Islands.

Appendix C

General Assistance, General Medical Assistance, and Emergency Assistance, by State

	State General Assistance for Those "Pending SSI" or Who "Only" Have ARC		
State	*Welfare Payments*	*Medical Assistance*	*Emergency Assistance*[1]
AL	None	None*	None
AK	Yes	Yes	None
AZ	Urban areas[3]	Yes	Limited[2]
AR	None	None*	None
CA	Yes	Yes	Yes
CO	Urban areas[3]	Yes	Urban areas[3]
CT	Yes	Yes	Yes
DE	Urban areas[3]	None*	Yes
DC	Yes	Yes	Yes
FL	Urban areas[3]	Yes	Urban areas[3]
GA	Yes[4]	None*	None
HI	Yes	Yes	Yes
ID	None	Yes	Limited[2]
IL	Yes	Yes	Yes
IN	None	None*	None
IA	Yes	None*	Urban areas[3]
KS	Yes[4]	Yes	Urban areas[3]
KY	Yes[4]	None*	None
LA	None	None*	None
ME	None	Yes	Urban areas[3]
MD	Yes	Yes	Yes[2]
MA	Yes	Yes	Yes
MI	Yes	Yes	Yes
MN	Yes	Yes	Yes
MS	None	None*	None
MO	Yes	Yes	Urban areas[3]
MT	Yes[4]	Yes	None
NE	Yes[4]	Some counties[3]*	Yes
NV	None	Yes	None

State General Assistance for Those
"Pending SSI" or Who "Only"
Have ARC

State	Welfare Payments	Medical Assistance	Emergency Assistance[1]
NH	Yes[4]	None*	None
NJ	Yes	Yes	Yes
NM	None	None*	Limited[2]
NY	Yes	Yes	Yes
NC	Yes[4]	None*	None
ND	None	Some counties[3]*	None
OH	Yes	Yes	Urban areas[3]
OK	None	None*	None
OR	Yes[4]	Yes	Yes
PA	Yes	Yes	Yes
RI	Yes	Yes	Yes
SC	None	None*	None
SD	None	Some counties[3]*	None
TN	Yes[4]	None*	None
TX	None	Yes	None
UT	Yes[4]	Yes	None
VT	Yes	Yes	Yes
VA	Urban areas[3]	Urban areas[3]*	None
WA	Yes	Yes	Yes
WV	None	None*	Yes
WI	Yes	Yes	Yes
WY	None	Yes	None

Source: Adapted by author from data reported by states to the Social Security Administration, as of mid-1989, as well as from Patricia Butler's *Too Poor To Be Sick* (1989) and reports of the Intergovernmental Health Policy Project of George Washington University.

[1] At least some minimal Emergency Assistance is available in all states for families with children; this listing, however, is for Emergency Assistance programs for the *childless disabled*.

[2] Statewide Emergency Assistance program subject to dollar limit per case, or provides only limited services (such as prevention of eviction), or both.

[3] Because state program is partially or fully funded by individual counties, only more liberal areas provide services.

[4] General Assistance cash welfare payments may be limited to those actually awaiting SSI eligibility decision, and thus not be available to others (such as those already found "not disabled enough" for SSI).

* Free or reduced-fee medical care for indigents may be available at city, county, state, or state university hospitals or clinics. Apply at registration or business office.

Note: General Medical Assistance for those poor who do not (yet) meet the SSDI/SSI definition of disability is usually more limited than that offered under the federal Medicaid program; access might be limited to public hospitals or clinics, or might only be covered on a funds-available, treatment-by-treatment basis, or might be limited only to emergency inpatient hospital care. On the other hand, a few liberal, urban states' General Medical Assistance is essentially the same as Medicaid. Apply at the local welfare office, or at the registration or business office of the public hospital or clinic.

Appendix D

SSDI/SSI Medical Disability for AIDS and ARC

C O N T E N T S

Note: Reproduction of appendices D–2a, D–2b, D–3a, D–3b, D–4, and D–5, adapted from Patrick James' *Guide for Social Security Disability Insurance Claims for HIV Disease—AIDS-ARC*, by permission of Aids Benefits Counselors (1547 California Street, San Francisco, CA 94109), is permitted free if it is to go to persons with AIDS or ARC without charge, in accordance with the wishes of the deceased author.

4 Claimant/Physician Functional Capacity Report (Adapted from James' *Guide for SSDI Claims*)

5 Daily Activities Questionnaire: Third Party Information (Adapted from James' *Guide for SSDI Claims*)

6 Coping with the Social Security Disability Determination Process

24525.000 Evaluation of Acquired Immunodeficiency Syndrome (AIDS) and AIDS-Related Complex (ARC)

MEDICAL EVALUATION

TN 10 9-87 DI 24525.001B.

Evaluation of Acquired Immunodeficiency Syndrome (AIDS) and AIDS-Related Complex (ARC)

24525.001 Criteria for Identifying AIDS

AIDS is characterized by defect in natural immunity against disease. It is caused by a specific retrovirus known as human immunodeficiency virus (HIV).

To meet or equal the Social Security Listing of Impairments, AIDS must be manifested by one or more diseases indicative of AIDS. Originally, diseases indicative of AIDS, based on available knowledge, ensured a reasonable predictive value for underlying immunodeficiency caused by what was then an unknown agent. The indicators of AIDS were restricted to particular opportunistic diseases diagnosed by reliable methods in individuals without specific known causes of immunodeficiency. After HIV was discovered to be the cause of AIDS, however, the spectrum of manifestations of HIV-infection became better defined, and it became apparent that some progressive and seriously disabling conditions were not included in the definition of AIDS.

The following criteria include severe HIV-associated conditions that are indicative of AIDS.

A. Without Laboratory Evidence Regarding HIV Infection

If laboratory tests for HIV were not performed or gave inconclusive results (See Exhibit A) and the individual had no other cause of immunodeficiency listed in Section A.1 below, then any disease listed in Section A.2 indicates AIDS if it was diagnosed by a definitive method (See Exhibit B).

1. Causes of immunodeficiency that disqualify diseases as indicators of AIDS in the absence of laboratory evidence for HIV infection

a. high-dose or long-term systemic corticosteriod therapy or other immunosuppresive/cytotoxic therapy within 3 months before the onset of the indicator disease

b. any of the following diseases diagnosed within 3 months after diagnosis of the indicator disease: Hodgkin's disease, non-Hodgkin's lymphoma (other than primary brain lymphoma), lymphocytic leukemia, multiple myeloma, any other cancer of lymphoreticular or histiocytic tissue, or angioimmunoblastic lymphadenopathy

c. a genetic (congenital) immunodeficiency syndrome or an acquired immunodeficiency syndrome atypical of HIV infection, such as one involving hypogammaglobulinemia

2. Indicator diseases diagnosed definitively (See Exhibit B)

a. candidiasis of the esophagus, trachea, bronchi, or lungs

b. cryptococcosis, extrapulmonary

c. cryptosporidiosis with diarrhea persisting over 1 month

d. cytomegalovirus disease of an organ other than liver, spleen, lymph nodes in an individual over 1 month of age

e. herpes simplex virus infection causing a mucocutaneous ulcer that persists longer than 1 month; or bronchitis, pneumonitis, or esophagitis for any duration affecting a individual over 1 month of age

f. Kaposi's sarcoma affecting an individual less than 60 years of age

g. lymphoma of the brain (primary) affecting an individual less than 60 years of age

h. lymphoid interstitial pneumonia and/or pulmonary lymphoid hyperplasia (LIP/PLH complex) affecting a child less than 13 years of age

i. mycobacterium avium complex or M. kansasii disease, disseminated (at a site other than or in addition to lungs, skin, or cervical or hilar lymph nodes)

j. pneumocystis carinii pneumonia

k. progressive multifocal leukoencephalopathy

l. toxoplasmosis of the brain affecting an individual over 1 month of age

B. With Laboratory Evidence for HIV Infection

Regardless of the presence of other causes of immunodeficiency (A.1) in the presence of laboratory evidence of HIV infection (See Exhibit A), any disease listed above (A.2) or below (B.1 or B.2) indicates a diagnosis of AIDS.

1. Indicator diseases diagnosed definitively (See Exhibit B)

a. bacterial infections, multiple or recurrent (any combination of at least two within a 2-year period), of the following types affecting a child less than 13 years of age:

septicemia, pneumonia, meningitis, bone or joint infection, or abscess of an internal organ or body cavity (excluding otitis media or superficial skin or mucosal abscesses), caused by Haemophilus, Streptococcus (including pneumococcus), or other pyogenic bacteria

b. coccidioidomycosis, disseminated (at a site other than or in addition to lungs or cervical or hilar lymph nodes)

c. HIV encephalopathy (also called "HIV dementia," "AIDS dementia," or "subacute encephalitis due to HIV") (See Exhibit B for description)

d. histoplasmosis, disseminated (at a site other than or in addition to lungs or cervical or hilar lymph nodes)

e. isosporiasis with diarrhea persisting over 1 month

f. Kaposi's sarcoma at any age

g. lymphoma of the brain (primary) at any age

h. other non-Hodgkin's lymphoma of B-cell or unknown immunologic phenotype and the following histologic types:

— small noncleaved lymphoma (either Burkitt or non-Burkitt type)

— immunoblastic sarcoma (equivalent to any of the following, although not necessarily all in combination: immunoblastic lymphoma, large-cell lymphoma, diffuse histiocytic lymphoma, diffuse undifferentiated lymphoma, or high-grade lymphoma)

NOTE: *Lymphomas are not included here if they are of T-cell immunologic phenotype or their histologic type is not described or is described as "lymphocyctic," "lymphoblastic," "small cleaved," or "plasmacytoid lymphocytic"*

i. any mycobacterial disease caused by mycobacteria other than M. tuberculosis, disseminated (at a site other than or in addition to lungs, skin, or cervical or hilar lymph nodes)

j. disease caused by M. tuberculosis, extrapulmonary (involving at least one site outside the lungs, regardless of whether there is concurrent pulmonary involvement)

k. salmonella (nontyphoid) septicemia, recurrent

l. HIV wasting syndrome (emaciation, "slim disease") (See Exhibit B for description)

2. Indicator disease diagnosed presumptively (by a method other than those in Exhibit B)

NOTE: *Given the seriousness of diseases indicative of AIDS, it is generally important to diagnose them definitively. Nonetheless, in some situations, an individual's condition will not permit the performance of definitive tests. In other situations, accepted clinical practice may be to diagnose presumptively based on the presence of characteristic clinical and laboratory abnormalities. Suggested guidelines used for presumptive diagnosis are in Exhibit C.*

a. candidiasis of the esophagus

b. cytomegalovirus retinitis with loss of vision

c. Kaposi's sarcoma

d. lymphoid interstitial pneumonia and/or pulmonary lymphoid hyperplasia (LIP/PLH complex) affecting a child less than 13 years of age

e. mycobacterial disease (acid-fast bacilli with species not identified by culture), disseminated (involving at least one site other than or in addition to lungs, skin, or cervical or hilar lymph nodes)

f. pneumocystis carinii pneumonia

g. toxoplasmosis of the brain affecting an individual over 1 month of age

C. With Laboratory Evidence Against HIV Infection

With laboratory test results negative for HIV infection (See Exhibit A), a diagnosis of AIDS is ruled out unless:

1. all the other causes of immunodeficiency listed above in Section A.1 are excluded; AND

2. the patient has had either:

a. pneumocystis carinii pneumonia diagnosed by a definitive method (See Exhibit B); OR

b. any of the other diseases indicative of AIDS listed above in Section A.2 diagnosed by a definitive method (See Exhibit B); AND a T-helper/inducer (CD4) lymphocyte count less than 400/mm².

While the foregoing criteria identify cases involving the more severe manifestations of AIDS, it does not describe the full spectrum of diseases seen in individuals who are believed to have a disease process resulting from the AIDS etiological agent, i.e., a disease moderately predictive of a defect in cell mediated immunity and there is no known cause of diminished resistance to that disease. Informed medical judgment must be exercised to determine whether other infections or diseases carry a level of severity and prognosis which is equivalent to the criteria described above. See DI 24525.010 for documentation requirements in such cases.

24525.005 AIDS-Related Complex (ARC)

In addition to AIDS as described in DI 24525.001, clinicians have identified a group of individuals with a variety of signs and symptoms which are thought to be caused by the virus HIV. These individuals commonly have some of the following findings: Recurrent fevers, lymphadenopathy, prolonged diarrhea, fatigue, weight loss, night sweats, recurrent fungal, viral, or other infections such as oral candidiasis. Some common laboratory findings may include: Positive antibody test for HIV, lymphopenia, T-cell reduction, T-cell ratio reversal or skin anergy. A variety of names have been used to identify this constellation of symptoms and signs including AIDS prodrome, generalized lymphadenopathy syndrome, pre-AIDS (no longer used), and AIDS-related complex (ARC). The latter term is now commonly used, though there is no universally accepted definition of this term at this time.

24525.010 Documentation of AIDS/ARC

The medical file should be documented by the findings of a thorough history and physical examination. Onset and the nature of signs and symptoms should be specifically and clearly described. Attempts should be made to quantify the extent and severity of all signs and symptoms. The variability or intensity of signs, symptoms and laboratory findings over time should also be indicated. It will often be necessary to obtain a detailed description of daily activities to describe functional limitations or abilities for those cases which require an assessment of RFC. Laboratory data of record providing the results of serological testing (including AIDS antibody, antigen or virus testing), microbiologic cultures, or tissue biopsy should also be obtained. However, in obtaining information regarding HIV antibody or viral testing DDS's should adhere to State and local laws governing the release of information.

While certain documentation of AIDS/ARC is desirable, it is not essential and should not be purchased. Included in this category are (1) HIV antibody or viral testing and (2) documentation of immune deficiency such an lymphocyte subpopulation study results.

When such tests are not part of the medical evidence of record, for Social Security disability purposes, a diagnosis of AIDS can be accepted if the individual has a disease moderately predictive of a defect in cell mediated immunity, and there is no known cause of diminished resistance to that disease. In such cases, the disease or opportunistic infection must be adequately documented by results of serological testing, microbiologic cultures, or tissue biopsy. Also, full details of the claimant's history and clinical course relative to the AIDS syndrome must be documented.

24525.015 Evaluation of AIDS/ARC

The criteria in DI 24525.001 describe the most commonly occurring disease in individuals with AIDS and delineate a population of individuals who have recurrent life-threatening illnesses which impose severe functional limitations and have a mortality rate approaching 100 percent. Therefore, once an individual has a confirmed diagnosis of AIDS, and is not engaging in substantial gainful activity, the level of severity of the individual's impairment will be considered to meet or equal the Listing of Impairments in appendix 1, subpart P of Regulations No. 4. Thus, a documented case of AIDS will be found to meet any applicable listed impairment or to be medically equivalent to any closely related listed impairment.

Because of the known high mortality rate in AIDS cases, for purposes of duration, that aspect of the definition of disability, "expected to result in death," would be applicable to an individual with AIDS. Therefore, due to the prognosis of death, an individual with documented AIDS would meet the duration requirement under sections 404.1509 and 416.909 of the regulations. As long as an individual with AIDS is not engaging in substantial gainful activity (SGA) (sections 404.1520(b) and 416.920(b)), he or she will be found to be under a disability under sections 404.1520(d), 404.1578 (widows, widowers, and surviving divorced spouses), 416.920(d) and 416.906 (title XVI children) of the regulations.

Those individuals who do not meet the criteria in DI 24525.001, but who have evidence of AIDS/ARC should not automatically be assumed to have an impairment which does not meet or equal the listings. Such individuals' claims must be assessed on a case-by-case basis. As with all medically determinable impairments, the assessment of severity must take into account signs, symptoms, and laboratory findings. Development and assessment of activities of daily living may also be helpful in evaluating the severity of the impairment. If the listings are not met or equaled, these cases should be sequentially evaluated.

Many individuals with AIDS/ARC present with signs and symptoms suggesting a mental impairment, e.g., organic mental disorder, depression, etc. In such cases, the nature and severity of any mental impairment should be fully developed, including, if necessary, an assessment of mental RFC.

In certain ARC cases, when there has been a recent onset, it may be appropriate to defer adjudication. However, this should be done with discretion so the message that SSA expects the impairment to become AIDS or disabling ARC is not conveyed.

24525.020 Onset of Disability

Onset of disability should be based on allegations, work history and the medical and other evidence concerning impairment severity (DI 25501.001 ff). Onset in cases of AIDS or ARC will be no later than the date medical findings show that the impairment is disabling unless the individual is engaging in SGA. These findings must include medical reports showing treatment for severe illness which could reasonably be attributed to the AIDS etiological agent and considered to represent a disabling impairment. In cases that meet the Social Security criteria for AIDS (DI 24525.001), the onset would be no later than the date of diagnosis unless the individual is engaging in SGA.

An earlier onset date of disability may be established if this is supported by the documented findings in the case. In some cases, it is reasonable to infer that the onset occurred some time prior to the first recorded medical examination, provided the claimant was not engaging in SGA. (See DI 25501.015.) However, an automatic date (e.g., 6 months prior to medical evidence) should not be inferred; the inference must be made based on all of the facts in each individual case.

24525.025 Diagnosis Coding

For an AIDS case to meet or equal a listing, there must be a diagnosis of AIDS plus a diagnosis of one of the diseases that indicate AIDS. The primary diagnosis in all AIDS cases should be 0420. In addition, the specific indicator disease should be coded as the secondary diagnosis. (See DI 27015.065.) The primary diagnosis in ARC cases should be 0430. Any secondary diagnosis in an ARC case also should be shown.

24525.030 Routing of Case Material

The DDS should forward a photocopy of the SSA-831-U5 only for AIDS cases which are allowed as meeting the definition of AIDS to the Office of Medical Evaluation (OME). However, the DDS should forward a photocopy of all case material for all AIDS cases that are denied and all ARC cases allowed or denied. So that OME will know when a disability quality branch (DQB) has revised a DDS decision, the DQB's should also forward photocopies of any revised SSA-831-U4, SSA-1774-U4(s), and any new medical evidence for all AIDS/ARC cases which they return. The case material should be sent to the Office of Medical Evaluation, Room 2030 Dickinson Building, 1500 Woodlawn Drive, Baltimore, Maryland 21241.

24525.035 Reexam Diaries

A 7-year medical improvement not expected (MINE) diary should be established on AIDS cases that meet the Social Security criteria and the MINE/permanent impairment listing code 241 should be used. However, until mortality experience with ARC cases is documented, a 3-year medical improvement possible (MIP) diary should be established for all ARC cases.

All ARC cases must be listed in item 26 (List No.) of the SSA-831-U5 using code 511. The identification will permit the retrieval of these cases for further study.

24525.095 Exhibits

Exhibit A

Laboratory Evidence For or Against HIV Infection

1. For Infection:
    When an individual has disease consistent with AIDS:
    a. a serum specimen from an individual 15 months of age or older, or from a child less than 15 months of age whose mother is not thought to have had HIV infection during the child's perinatal period, that is repeatedly reactive for HIV antibody by a screening test (e.g., enzyme-linked immunosorbent assay ([ELISA]), as long as subsequent HIV-antibody tests (e.g., Western blot, immunofluorescence assay), if done, are positive; OR
    b. a serum specimen from a child less than 15 months of age, whose mother is thought to have had HIV infection during the child's perinatal period, that is repeatedly reactive for HIV antibody by a screening test (e.g., ELISA), plus increased serum immunoglobulin levels and at least one of the following abnormal immunologic test results: reduced absolute lymphocyte count, depressed CD4 (T-helper) lymphocyte count, or decreased CD4/CD8 (helper/suppressor) ratio, as long as subsequent antibody tests (e.g., Western blot, immunofluorescence assay), if done, are positive; OR
    c. a positive test for HIV serum antigen; OR
    d. a positive HIV culture confirmed by both reverse transcriptase detection and a specific HIV-antigen test or in situ hybridization using a nucleic acid probe; OR
    e. a positive result on any other highly specific test for HIV (e.g., nucleic acid probe of peripheral blood lymphocytes).
2. Against Infection:
    A nonreactive screening test for serum antibody to HIV (e.g., ELISA) without a reactive or positive result on any other test for HIV infection (e.g., antibody, antigen, culture), if done.
3. Inconclusive (Neither For nor Against Infection):
    a. a repeatedly reactive screening test for serum antibody to HIV (e.g., ELISA) followed by a negative or inconclusive supplemental test (e.g., Western blot, immunofluorescence assay) without a positive HIV culture or serum antigen test, if done; OR
    b. a serum specimen from a child less than 15 months of age, whose mother is thought to have had HIV infection during the child's perinatal period, that is repeatedly reactive for HIV antibody by a screening test, even if positive by a supplemental test, without additional evidence for immunodeficiency as described above (in 1.b) and without a positive HIV culture or serum antigen test, if done.

Exhibit B

Definitive Diagnostic Methods for Diseases Indicative of AIDS

Diseases   **Definitive Diagnostic Methods**

cryptosporidiosis
cytomegalovirus
isosporiasis
Kaposi's sarcoma
lymphoma
lymphoid pneumonia or hyperplasia   microscopy (histology or cytology)
pneumocystis carinii pneumonia
progressive multifocal leukoencephalopathy
toxoplasmosis

candidiasis   gross inspection by endoscopy or autopsy or by microscopy
                                                (histology or cytology) on a specimen obtained directly from
                                                the tissues affected (including scrapings from the mucosal
                                                surface), not from a culture.

coccidioidomycosis   microscopy (histology or cytology), culture, or detection of
cryptococcosis   antigen in a specimen obtained directly from the tissues
herpes simplex virus   affected or a fluid from those tissues.
histoplasmosis

tuberculosis
other mycobacteriosis
salmonellosis   culture
other bacterial infection

HIV encephalopathy (dementia)   clinical findings of disabling cognitive and/or motor dysfunc-
                                                tion interfering with occupation or activities of daily living,
                                                or loss of behavioral developmental milestones affecting a
                                                child, progressing over weeks to months, in the absence of a
                                                concurrent illness or condition other than HIV infection that
                                                could explain such findings. Methods to rule out such concur-
                                                rent illnesses and conditions must include cerebrospinal fluid
                                                examination and either brain imaging (computed tomography
                                                or magnetic resonance) or autopsy.

HIV wasting syndrome   findings of profound involuntary weight loss (more than 10
                                                percent of baseline body weight) plus either chronic diarrhea
                                                (2 or more loose stools per day for 30 days or more) or
                                                chronic weakness and documented fever (for 30 days or
                                                more, intermittent or constant) in the absence of a concurrent
                                                illness or condition other than HIV infection that could
                                                explain the findings (e.g., cancer, tuberculosis, cryptospori-
                                                diosis or other specific enteritis).

DI 24525.095 (Cont.)   TN 10 9-87

Exhibit C

Suggested Guidelines for Presumptive Diagnosis of Disease Indicative of AIDS

Diseases	Presumptive Diagnostic Criteria
candidiasis of esophagus	a. recent onset of retrosternal pain on swallowing; AND b. oral candidiasis diagnosed by the gross appearance of white patches or plaques on an erythematous base or by the microscopic appearance of fungal mycelial filaments in an uncultured specimen scraped from the oral mucosa.
cytomegalovirus retinitis	a characteristic appearance on serial ophthalmoscopic examinations (e.g., discrete patches of retinal whitening with distinct borders, spreading in a centrifugal manner, following blood vessels, progressing over several months, frequently associated with retinal vasculitis, hemorrhage, and necrosis). Resolution of active disease leaves retinal scarring and atrophy with retinal pigment epithelial mottling.
mycobacteriosis	microscopy of a specimen from stool or normally sterile body fluids or tissue from a site other than lungs, skin, or cervical or hilar lymph nodes, showing acid-fast bacilli of a species not identified by culture.
Kaposi's sarcoma	a characteristic gross appearance of an erythematous or violaceous plaque-like lesion on skin or mucous membrane. (NOTE *Presumptive diagnosis of Kaposi's sarcoma should not be made by clinicians who have seen few cases of it.*)
lymphoid interstitial pneumonia	bilateral reticulonodular interstitial pulmonary infiltrates present on chest X ray for 2 months or more with no pathogen identified and no response to antibiotic treatment.
pneumocystis carinii pneumonia	a. a history of dyspnea on exertion or nonproductive cough of recent onset (within the past 3 months); AND b. chest X-ray evidence of diffuse bilateral interstitial infiltrates or gallium scan evidence of diffuse bilateral pulmonary disease; AND c. arterial blood gas analysis showing an arterial pO2 of less than 70 mm Hg or a low respiratory diffusing capacity (less than 80 percent of predicted values) or an increase in the alveolar-arterial oxygen tension gradient; AND d. no evidence of a bacterial pneumonia.
toxoplasmosis of the brain	a. recent onset of a focal neurologic abnormality consistent with intracranial disease or a reduced level of consciousness; AND b. brain imaging evidence of a lesion having a mass effect (on computed tomography or nuclear magnetic resonance) or the radiographic appearance of which is enhanced by injection of contrast medium; AND c. serum antibody to toxoplasmosis or successful response to therapy for toxoplasmosis.

PROVIDING MEDICAL EVIDENCE
FOR INDIVIDUALS WITH AIDS AND ARC

A Guide for Health Professionals
by the Social Security Administration

The following guidelines were developed to assist health professionals in providing the Social Security Administration with the type of medical evidence necessary for a disability claim decision for persons with AIDS or ARC. While these guidelines are not inclusive of every possible symptom or finding, they should assist you in documenting the disabled individual's condition adequately for Social Security purposes.   We appreciate your cooperation in providing complete reports.

Evaluation of Acquired Immunodeficiency Syndrome

Under the law, to be considered disabled for Social Security purposes, a person must be unable to do any substantial gainful work because of a medical condition which has lasted or is expected to last for at least 12 months or to end in death. People who have acquired immunodeficiency syndrome (AIDS) ordinarily will be severely limited in their ability to work and are unlikely to recover. Therefore, if the evidence shows that a person has AIDS, (as described by the Centers for Disease Control effective September 1, 1987), is not working, and meets other requirements for entitlement, he or she will be found disabled for Social Security purposes.

Evaluation of AIDS-Related Complex

Some people with ARC are unable to work and, therefore, are eligible for benefits if they meet the other requirements for entitlement to Social Security disability benefits. However, others with ARC may be less impaired. Therefore, all of the symptoms, signs and laboratory findings are evaluated on a case-by-case basis to determine the person's capacity for work functions. If a determination of disability cannot be made on medical grounds alone, then a determination is based on whether the claimant can do work he or she has done in the past or whether, considering the vocational factors of age, education and work experience, he or she can do other work.

SSA/SFRO/DPB
7/88

PREPARING THE MEDICAL REPORT

The medical evidence required for the adjudication of AIDS/ARC cases is similar to that required for all medical conditions. The evidence must be sufficiently complete to permit an independent determination by the DDS medical consultant as to the nature and limiting effects of the individual's physical or mental impairment and the probable duration of impairment.

History
Reports should include a thorough history which emphasizes the onset of the claimant's illness. It is important to describe the longitudinal course of the illness emphasizing the severity of signs and symptom over time to aid in determining when the illness became disabling.   While individuals with a documented AIDS diagnosis will be allowed on a medical basis, they may be eligible for an earlier onset due to the severity of their disease prior to the AIDS diagnosis.   Establishing the correct onset date is important not only for determining if and when disability criteria are met, but also affect when cash benefits and Medicare may begin. Quantification of duration and severity of all symptoms and signs is particularly important in the history. A description of limitation of function which results from the claimant's illness is very important. For example, a description of what activities the claimant can or cannot do as a result of fatigue, pain, mental changes, or other symptoms and signs is an important indicator of the severity of impairment.

Findings, Diagnosis, Prognosis
The report should describe the findings of a thorough physical examination documenting standard positive and negative findings.   Progress notes that document physical findings are particularly useful, but are not a substitute for a complete physical exam.

Copies of laboratory findings should be included as well as HIV testing results if they are available. (The State Disability Determination Service which evaluates disability claims for SSA has available an appropriate release form for HIV test results in California.)

A diagnosis and prognosis should be provided which are supported by the medical data.

Assessment of Work-Related Activities
Finally, the medical report should provide an assessment of the claimant's ability to do work-related activities such as sitting, standing, moving about, lifting, carrying, handling objects, hearing, speaking, and traveling and in the case of a mental impairment, the ability to reason or make occupational personal or social adjustments.

The physician may refer to the following outline which describes the type of information which is particularly useful to SSA. These findings represent frequently encountered changes due to HIV infection, but are by no means an exhaustive list.   Both normal and abnormal findings should be described. Fluctuations or changes in signs, symptoms or laboratory findings over time should be documented to assist in determining severity and duration of disability.

SYMPTOMS OF AIDS/ARC

1. Low energy, easy fatiguability, generalized weakness

2. Fevers/night sweats

3. Weight loss

4. Dyspnea on exertion

5. Persistent cough

6. Persistent diarrhea

7. Depression/anxiety

8. Forgetfulness, loss of concentration and slowness of thought

9. Other symptoms such as headache, anorexia, nausea, vomiting and rash (consider possible drug side effects as many patients are taking antiviral agents, immune modulators, or other medications which have serious side-effects.

SIGNS OF AIDS/ARC

1. Documented weight loss

2   Documented fevers

3. Lymphadenopathy

4. Oral thrush and/or hairy leukoplakia

5. Abnormal skin conditions

6. Asthenia

7. Depression or other mental changes

8. Central or peripheral neurologic deficit

SSA/SFRO/DPB
7/88

LABORATORY ABNORMALITIES

1. Leukopenia, lymphopenia, anemia or thrombocytopenia

2. Elevated sedimentation rate

3. Elevated serum globulins

4. Depressed helper T-cell Count

5. Inverted helper/suppressor ratio

6. Positive HIV antibody test (including confirmatory test)

7. X-ray or imaging changes

8. Microbiology and pathology reports

9. Other indicators of immune status such as elevated beta-2-microglobulins, detectable p24 antigen, etc.

DESCRIPTION OF FUNCTIONAL LIMITATIONS

1. Ability (or limitation in ability) to independently bathe, dress, shop, cook, drive, or take public transportation

2. Ability (or limitation in ability) to perform specific activities such as carrying a 15 pound bag of groceries up a flight of stairs

3. Ability (or limitation in ability) to stand/walk for 6-8 hours per day and ability to sit for 6-8 hours per day.

4. Ability (or limitation in ability) to reason, concentrate or perform other mental tasks

5. Ability (or limitation in ability) in any other areas that might affect the claimant's potential for work related activities.

NOTE: The more specific the details of abilities and limitations, the easier it is to make a sound decision.

Department of Health and Human Services

Social Security Administration

20 CFR Part 416

[Regulations No. 16]
Supplemental Security Income for the
Aged, Blind, and Disabled;
Presumptive Disability and
Presumptive Blindness; Categories of
Impairments—AIDS

Agency: Social Security Administration. HHS.
Action: Final rule

Summary: We may pay benefits to a person applying for supplemental security income benefits on the basis of disability or blindness before making a formal determination when available information indicates a high probability that disability exists. These findings of presumptive disability and blindness may be made at the Social Security district offices only for specified impairment categories; at the State agencies, they may be made for any impairment category. We are publishing final rules which add acquired immunodeficiency syndrome (AIDS) to these categories in view of the predictability that the disease will result in a finding of disability.

Date: Effective February 9, 1988. These final regulations will be effective through December 31, 1989, when they will expire, unless extended or revised and promulgated again.[1]

For Further Information Contact: William J. Ziegler, Legal Assistant, Office of Regulations, Social Security Administration, 6401 Security Boulevard, Baltimore, MD 21235, Telephone (301) 965-1759.

Supplementary Information: Section 1631(a)(4)(B) of the Social Security Act (the Act) provides that a claimant applying for supplemental security income benefits based on disability or blindness may receive up to 3 months' payments prior to the determination of the individual's disability or blindness if he or she is presumptively disabled or blind and otherwise eligible. Any such payments based on presumptive disability or blindness are not considered overpayments if it is later determined that the person is not disabled or blind, unless the person is disallowed benefits due to a nondisability eligibility criterion or it is later determined that the amount of the payment was incorrectly calculated.

A finding of presumptive disability or presumptive blindness is made at the district office in cases where the available evidence or other information, including observations and confirming contacts, indicates a high degree of probability that the claimant is disabled or blind, even though the evidence may be insufficient for a final determination of disability or blindness by the State agency.

A State agency may also make a finding of presumptive disability or blindness. Generally, a presumptive finding of disability or blindness made at the State agency may be based on any impairment when the evidence is sufficient to determine that there is a high degree of probability that the finding will later be confirmed when complete evidence is obtained.

On the other hand, district office findings are restricted to impairment categories for which experience has shown that particularly reliable findings of presumptive disability and presumptive blindness can be made. The district office may find presumptive disability and blindness in those situations specified in 20 CFR 416.934, provided that the claimant's statements about his or her medical condition are consistent with observations of the district office representative or supported by confirming contacts. These limitations insure that presumptive findings are seldom reversed when actual medical evidence is considered for the formal disability or blindness determinations by the State agency.

On February 11, 1985, we published interim regulations in the **Federal Register** (50 FR 5573) adding AIDS as then defined by the Centers for Disease Control (CDC) to the impairment categories in § 416.934 to permit district offices to find presumptive disability for this disease. These regulations were effective February 11, 1985.

Under the final regulations, the district office may find presumptive disability when a claimant, who is not working, alleges disability due to AIDS after a confirming contact has been made to ascertain that this disease with one or more manifestations (described in Appendix 1 of Subpart I) has been diagnosed by a licensed physician. Confirmation of this diagnosis will be by contact with a physician or some other medical or treating source, such as a member of a hospital or clinic staff who is able to confirm that such a diagnosis has been made. This confirming contact may be made by telephone. Presumptive disability may be found immediately upon confirmation of the diagnosis of AIDS with manifestation(s) in Appendix 1 and need not be delayed for the receipt of the actual medical reports or records. A final disability determination will be made later when sufficient medical evidence is received by the State agency.

We are extending the expiration date in these final regulations. This presumptive disability category for AIDS will be effective through December 31, 1989. Several treatments are now being tested, and additional time is needed to be able to evaluate the efficacy of these treatments. Because of the dynamic nature of research concerning the diagnosis, evaluation, and treatment of AIDS, this impairment category will require periodic review and reassessment. We intend to carefully monitor these regulations by providing for ongoing evaluation of the impairment category to determine whether they will need to be revised and updated to reflect advancements in scientific knowledge and treatment of this disease. Therefore, these final regulations will cease to be effective after December 31, 1989, unless extended by the Secretary or revised and promulgated again as a result of the findings from the evaluation period.[1]

Public Comments

Interested persons, organizations, and groups were invited to submit data, views or arguments pertaining to the interim regulations within a period of 60 days from the date of publication. The comment period ended on April 12, 1985. Following are our responses to the comments.

Comment: One commenter indicated that the CDC's definition of AIDS was formulated for the purpose of epidemiologic surveillance and that it may be too "restrictive" to use in determining presumptive disability. The commenter expressed concern that use of that definition may exclude claimants who are disabled, despite their not meeting the specific criteria of the CDC definition.

We did not think at the time the interim regulations were published that CDC's definition was too restrictive for the district offices to use in determining presumptive disability because, when a presumptive disability decision is made, it must be highly probable that disability will be found later when the medical evidence is obtained. We have also reviewed the revised CDC surveillance definition of AIDS (effective September 1, 1987) which defines AIDS in terms of its manifestation(s) by certain indicator diseases, including human immunodeficiency virus (HIV) encephalopathy ("HIV dementia") and HIV wasting syndrome. We have determined that individuals who meet the revised definition and are not working may be found to be presumptively disabled for Social Security purposes.

However, we agree that the CDC definition of AIDS should not be directly linked to Social Security presumptive disability determinations. CDC and SSA view AIDS from different perspectives. CDC defines AIDS for public health and other purposes that are not necessarily intended to have prognostic significance nor to designate the severity of the illness. By contrast, SSA must determine if the presumptive disability requirements of the law are met. Moreover, SSA has no control over possible future revisions of the CDC definition and uses no other program controlled definition or criteria to establish SSA presumptive disability eligibility. Therefore, although we have deleted specific reference to the CDC definition of AIDS form the regulations, we are incorporating, for purposes of these regulations, the criteria of the September 1, 1987 CDC definition of AIDS cases into the regulations in Appendix 1. The net effect of this change is two-fold: It includes in the regulations all the AIDS cases that meet the criteria of the CDC definition effective September 1, 1987, but it also means that future revisions to the CDC definition of AIDS will not automatically affect SSA presumptive disability determinations. However, we will look closely at any such revisions and, if appropriate for presumptive disability purposes, we will modify our eligibility criteria accordingly.

Comment: One commenter objected to the statement in the preamble to the intermim rule that the district office confirm with a medical or treating source that the disease has progressed to the point that the individual is unable to work. This commenter believed that once the CDC definition of AIDS has been diagnosed, it would be redundant to ask if the claimant has the physical capacity to work.

Response: We agree with the comment. We believe that it is highly unlikely that an individual with AIDS that meets the CDC definition either before, or as of, September 1, 1987 would be able to engage in substantial gainful activity. Therefore, for purposes of making the presumptive disability decision, it would be unnecesssary to ask the treating source for an opinion regarding the individual's ability to work.

Other comments expressed favorable views about these regulations.

Regulatory Procedures
Executive Order 12291

The Secretary has determined that this is not a major rule under Executive Order 12291 because these regulations do not meet any of the threshold criteria for a major rule. Therefore, a regulatory impact analysis is not required.

Regulatory Flexibily Act

We certify that these regulations will not have a significant economic impact on a substantial number of small entities because they only affect a small number of disability claimants under Title XVI of the Social Security Act.

Paperwork Reduction Act

These regulations impose no reporting/recordkeeping requirements necessitating clearance by the Office of Management and Budget.

(Catalog of Federal Domestic Program No. 13.807, Supplemental Security Income Program)

List of Subjects in 20 CFR Part 416

Administrative practice and procedure, Aged, Blind, Disability benefits, Public assistance programs, Supplemental Security Income.

Dated: October 5, 1987.

Dorcas R. Hardy,
Commissioner of Social Security.
  Approval: December 4, 1987.

Otis R. Bowen,

Secretary of Health and Human Services.

For the reasons set out in the preamble, Part 416, Subpart I, Chapter III of Title 20, Code of Federal Regulations, is amended as set forth below.

**Part 416—Supplemental
Security Income for the Aged,
Blind, and Disabled**

Subpart I—Determining Disability and Blindness

1. The authority citation for Subpart I continues to read as follows:

Authority: Secs. 1102.1164(a), 1619, 1631(a) and (d)(1), and 1633 of the Social Security Act; 42 U.S.C. 1302 1382c(a), 1382h, 1383(a) and (d)(1), and 1383b; secs. 2, 5, 6, and 15 Pub. L. 98–460, 98 Stat. 1794, 1801, 1802, and 1808.

2. Section 416.934 is amended by revising the introductory paragraph and paragraph (k) to read as follows:

§416.934 Impairments which may warrant a finding of presumptive disability or presumptive blindness.

We may make findings of presumptive disability and presumptive blindness in specific impairment categories without obtaining any medical evidence. These specific impairment categories are—

•　　•　　•　　•　　•

(k) Allegation of acquired immunodeficiency syndrome (AIDS) with one or more manifestations listed in Appendix 1 of this Subpart, as diagnosed by a licensed physician; this category is effective only through December 31, 1989, unless extended by the Secretary or revised and promulgated again.[1]

3. A new Appendix 1 is added to the end of Subpart I to read as follows:

Appendix 1 to Subpart I—Manifestations of Acquired Immunodeficiency Syndrome (AIDS)

I. Without Laboratory Evidence Regarding Human Immunodeficiency Virus (HIV) Infection

If laboratory tests for HIV were not performed or gave inconclusive results and the patient had no other cause of immunodeficiency listed in section I.A below, then any disease listed in section I.B indicates AIDS if it was diagnosed by a definitive method.

A. Causes of Immunodeficiency That Disqualify Diseases as Indicators of AIDS in the Absence of Laboratory Evidence for HIV Infection

1. High-dose or long-term systemic corticosteroid therapy or other immunosuppressive/cytotoxic therapy less than or equal to 3 months before the onset of the indicator disease.

2. Any of the following diseases diagnosed less than or equal to 3 months after diagnosis of the indicator disease: Hodgkin's disease, non-Hodgkin's lymphoma (other than primary brain lymphoma), lymphocytic leukemia, multiple myeloma, any other cancer of lymphoreticular or histiocytic tissues, or angioimmunoblastic lymphadenopathy.

3. A genetic (congential) immunodeficiency syndrome or an acquired immunodeficiency syndrome atypical of HIV infection, such as one involving hypogammaglobulinemia.

B. Indicator Diseases Diagnosed Definitively

1. Candidiasis of the esophagus, trachea, bronchi, or lungs.

2. Cryptococcosis, extrapulmonary.

3. Cryptosporidiosis with diarrhea persisting more than 1 month.

4. Cytomegalovirus disease of an organ other than liver, spleen, or lymph nodes in a patient more than 1 month of age.

5. Herpes simplex virus infection causing a mucocutaneous ulcer that persists more than 1 month, or bronchitis, pneumonitis, or esophagitis for any duration affecting a patient more than 1 month of age.

6. Kaposi's sarcoma affecting a patient under 60 years of age.

7. Lymphoma of the brain (primary) afecting a patient under 60 years of age.

8. Lymphoid interstitial pneumonia and/or pulmonary lymphoid hyperplasia (LIP/PLH complex) affecting a child under 13 years of age.

9. *Mycobacterium avium* complex or M. kansasii disease, disseminated (at a site other than or in addition to lungs, skin, or cervical or hilar lymph nodes).

10. *Pneumocystis carinii* pneumonia.

11. Progressive multifocal leukoencephalopathy.

12. Toxoplasmosis of the brain affecting a patient more than 1 month of age.

II. With Laboratory Evidence for HIV Infection

Regardless of the presence of other causes of immunodeficiency (I.A.), in the presence of laboratory evidence for HIV infection, any disease listed above (I.B.) or below (II.A or II.B) indicates a diagnosis of AIDS.

A. Indicator Diseases Diagnosed Definitively

1. Bacterial infections, multiple or recurrent (any combination of at least 2 within a 2-year period), of the following types affecting a child under 13 years of age:

Septicemia, pneumonia, meningitis, bone or joint infection, or abscess of an internal organ or body cavity (excluding otitis media or superficial skin or mucosal abscesses), caused by *Haemophilus, Streptococcus* (including pneumonococcus), or other pyogenic bacteria.

2. Coccidioidomycosis, disseminated (at a site other than or in addition to lungs or cervical or hilar lymph nodes).

3. HIV encephalopathy (also called "HIV dementia," "AIDS dementia," or "subacute encephalitis due to HIV").

4. Histoplasmosis, disseminated (at a site other than or in addition to lungs or cervical or hilar lymph nodes).

5. Isosporiasis with diarrhea persisting more than 1 month.

6. Kaposi's sarcoma at any age.

7. Lymphoma of the brain (primary) at any age.

8. Other non-Hodgkin's lymphoma of B-cell or unknown immunologic phenotype and the following histologic types:

a. Small noncleaved lymphoma (either Burkitt or non-Burkitt type).

b. Immunoblastic sarcoma (equivalent to any of the following, although not necessarily all in combination: immunoblastic lymphoma, large cell lymphoma, diffuse histiocytic lymphoma, diffuse undifferentiated lymphoma, or high-grade lymphoma).

Note: Lymphomas are not included here if they are of T-cell immunologic phenotype or their histologic type is not described or is described as "lymphocytic," "lymphoblastic," "small cleaved," or "plasmacytoid lymphocytic".

9. Any mycobacterial disease caused by mycobateria other than *M. tuberculosis,* disseminated (at a site other than or in addition to lungs, skin, or cervical or hilar lymph nodes).

10. Disease caused by *M. tuberculosis,* extrapulmonary (involving at least one site outside the lungs, regardless of whether there is concurrent pulmonary involvement).

11. *Salmonella* (nontyphoid) septicemia, reccurent.

12. HIV wasting syndrome (emaciation, "slim disease").

B. Indicator Disease Diagnosed Presumptively

Note: Given the seriousness of diseases indicative of AIDS, it is generally important to diagnose them definitively, especially when therapy that would be used may have serious side effects or when definitive diagnosis is needed for eligibility for antiretroviral therapy. Nonetheless, in some situations, a patient's condition will not permit the performance of definitive tests. In other situations, accepted clinical practice may be to diagnose presumptively based on the presence of characteristic clinical and laboratory abnormalities.

1. Candidiasis of the esophagus.

2. Cytomegalovirus retinitis with loss of vision.

3. Kaposi's sarcoma.

4. Lymphoid interstitial pneumonia and/or pulmonary lymphoid hyperplasia (LIP/PLH complex) affecting a child under 13 years of age.

5. Mycobacterial disease (acid-fast bacilli with species not identified by culture). disseminated (involving at least one site other than or in addition to lungs, skin, or cervical or hilar lymph nodes).

6. *Pneumocystis carinii* pneumonia.

7. Toxoplasmosis of the brain affecting a patient more than 1 month of age.

III. With Laboratory Evidence Against HIV Infection

With laboratory test results negative for HIV infection a diagnosis of AIDS is ruled out unless:

A. All the other causes of immunodeficiency listed above in section I.A are excluded; AND.

B. The patient has had either:

1. *Pneumocystis carinii* pneumonia diagnosed by a defintive method; OR.

2. a. Any of the other diseases indicative of AIDS listed above in section I.B diagnosed by a definitive method; AND.

b. A T-helper/inducer (CD4) lymphocyte count under 400/mm^3.

[FR Doc. 88–2722 Filed 2-8-88; 8:45 am].

Billing Code 4190–11–M

[1]Nevertheless, SSA will continue use of this regulation until the promulgation of a replacement.

ARC Disability for Social Security Benefits: Medical Report Instructions

The following evaluation form contains a list of major and minor clinical findings, immunologic and laboratory, that may result in disability for patients suffering from AIDS-Related Complex (ARC).

The points covered in this form may be stated in a narrative report and substituted. ARC patient claims are assessed on a case-by-case basis by Social Security. *It is important to stress how each finding is related to the patient's disability, ability to perform Substantial Gainful Activity (SGA, any type of work) and daily personal activities.* A statement of findings alone may not suffice to meet SSA Disability listings.

The symptoms and findings should indicate any variances observed over time.

Requirements to meet disability listings are generally *two* major clinical findings or *one* major finding and *two* or more minor findings. These should be accompanied by *one* or more Immunologic and *two* or more Laboratory findings.

Dementia and emaciation (wasting disorder) have been added as two disorders utilized to confirm an AIDS diagnosis by the federal Centers for Disease Control. The Social Security Administration adopted these findings as indicative of AIDS for the purpose of Presumptive Disability, effective 09/01/87. There is no anticipated expansion or variation from the previous SSA disability criteria for dementia or emaciation (wasting disorder—loss of 10% or more of body weight or 15 or more pounds). These disorders should be fully documented for ARC patients.

The Karnofsky Performance Status Scale has been attached to the format. To be considered disabled, a patient must have a score of 70 or less, "Cares for self, unable to carry on normal activity or do normal work."

The majority of ARC patient findings include severe diarrhea and fatigue. It is important to show the *severity* and *frequency* of these disorders (e.g., "needs immediate and continuous access to toilet facilities due to diarrhea"; "bed rest and frequent naps are required throughout the day due to fatigue"). It would be helpful to relate how these particular findings preclude normal work activity.

For Social Security purposes, the disability must be expected to last at least 12 months. A statement should be included in your report regarding the length of time the disability is expected to last.

A comprehensive narrative report for Social Security purposes should include the following:

- Medical history
- Longitudinal history
- Major and minor clinical findings
- Disabling factors of clinical findings
- Immunological findings
- Disabling factors of immunologic findings (if applicable)
- Patient's ability to perform any type of work as a result of findings and history: residual functional capacity (if any), i.e., ability to sit, stand, push, pull, etc.
- Any mental disorders or neurologic deficits observed
- Prognosis
- Length of time disability is expected to last

Sample Medical Narrative

The diagnosis is ARC. _____ is a 44-year-old white male who first complained to me of marked fatigue in May of 1987, and he stated that for the previous three months he had been having increasing trouble with fatigue and weakness. At that time he denied fevers or sweats. He complained of loose stools with some fecal urgency for the past six months and was usually having two or three stools per day and occasionally up to six stools per day, rarely with any blood. The patient knew that he was HIV antibody positive for probably the previous two years. In July of 1985, he told me that he was HIV antibody positive and that he had learned this relatively recently before that July 1985 visit. At that time he told me that he had had enlarged lymph nodes in the groin for the previous four months. He had had a right facial Bell's palsy while in Europe in March of 1985 and recovered within six weeks.

In the early part of 1987, when he began having the above-mentioned symptoms, we completed some immune parameters which included T-cell studies. On May 22, 1987, his T4 count was 168/cu. mm., with lower limit of normal being 518. At that time his white count was 3,700, his globulins were elevated, he had a mild elevation in the liver transaminases. He was found to have Endolimax nana in the stools and stool culture was negative. An exam at that point did not reveal any specific other focus for further workup.

At this time the patient wished to begin taking AZT, and based upon his HIV positive status and his T-cell values and his fatigue, he qualified for the criteria that were in place in July of 1987 for prescribing AZT. Through August, he was continuing to display the symptoms of fatigue and noted that he had his own upholstering business and was really having trouble working and focusing on his job. He said that he was really only able to work for very short periods of time and that he was becoming increasingly unable to work full time.

We applied for the AZT toward the end of August, and for some reason there was a prolonged period of time until authorization was received, and the patient ultimately began on September 11, 1987. His dosage has been 1200 mg. daily, and he has been fortunate enough to maintain the medication at that level since that time. He has tolerated the drug; however, it has not significantly improved his fatigue, and on October 9, 1987, he complained of continuing to feel profoundly fatigued and simply was not able to work sufficiently to support himself.

On October 23, I saw him and he complained of a two-week history of a nonproductive cough with dyspnea. He denied fevers and reported that night sweats that had been going on for some time were continuing. At this time he reported to me that he had cut down his work in 1985 to a 30-hour work week, but in January of 1987, had essentially not been working at all because of his fatigue, and had been living on his savings. He was too proud to tell me about this until just this visit on October 23, 1987. An examination on that day was not revealing of the specific cause for his cough. A chest X-ray showed faint interstitial parabronchial infiltrates. A sputum specimen was negative for Pneumocystis on that day and was also negative on the following day. A gallium pulmonary scan revealed diffuse uptake of gallium throughout both lung fields uniformly, which was compatible with a diagnosis of Pneumocystis. The patient was seen in pulmonary consultation with Dr. _____, who saw the patient in consultation and performed bronchoscopy. The bronchoscopy did not result in a diagnosis. The washings and biopsies were negative for Pneumocystis and negative for any inflammatory interstitial process.

The patient had been started on Septra Double Strength therapy empirically, and after the negative bronchoscopic findings on October 30, we discontinued the Septra. I switched him to Erythromycin and the cough began to be productive of a greenish sputum in one to two teaspoon amounts. It should be noted that by this time, November 3, he had had the cough almost a full month and it was now only starting to become productive. There was a nasal quality to his voice, and listening to his chest on November 3, there were scattered rhonchi throughout all lung fields. A tentative diagnosis of sinusitis and bronchitis was made and the feeling was that it was possibly secondary to bronchoscopy, and that a sputum should be obtained for culture and sensitivity and that the Erythromycin should be stopped and that a drug more compatible with nasopharyngeal pathogens should be started. Accordingly, he was started on Ceclor, 250 mg. t.i.d. for seven days. A chest X-ray was repeated and sputum was obtained for culture and sensitivity.

On the date of this dictation, November 16, two sputa have been obtained and they did not grow any abnormal pathogens. The patient's clinical status has been one of gradual improvement in his overall sense of well-being; however, his profound fatigue, of course, remains. A chest X-ray on November 10 shows persistent mild bibasilar interstitial and parabronchial lung densities. The patient's current clinical status is that of continued pulmonary infection, presumptive sinusitis and bronchitis. A sinus X-ray film series is pending. He continued on the Ceclor and his continued clinical course will be monitored carefully.

At this time the patient's status is felt to be compatible with the diagnosis of AIDS-related complex. It is clear that he is unable to work presently. It is hopeful that with continued maintenance on AZT he may regain strength sufficient to return to work, although he has been on that drug for three months and has not enjoyed an improvement to date. It is hoped that his previous clinical course can be illustrative of his course with ARC sufficiently to allow awarding of disability benefits to this patient. Disability is expected to last for at least 12 months.

Dictated by: _____, M.D.

Medical Evaluation Form

(Generic, nongovernment form to be submitted along with SSA's own forms to increase chance of being found "disabled"—especially useful in "ARC-only" cases.)

Patient Name

Social Security Number

Date Patient First Examined

Date of Most Recent Examination

Frequency of Visits

Onset Date of Disability
(This should not be today's date, or the date the patient first sought care from you or another practitioner, or even the date the patient first fully accepted the reality of his symptoms. Rather it is your best medical judgment as to the date—perhaps well in the past—when his disease first began preventing effective, ongoing work ability.)

This data should be based on allegations from patient, work history, medical discovery, or other discovery concerning severity of impairment.

CLINICAL FINDINGS

Major
Please state course of treatment and medication prescribed for each finding.

LYMPHADENOPATHY—Lymph nodes of 1 cm or more at 2 or more extrainguinal sites for at least 6 months (Note approximate size and locations)

ORAL THRUSH (Candida Albicans) (Note mucous membrane location(s), esophagus; state duration, recurrence after treatment)

HAIRY LEUKOPLAKIA (Note severity of infection and recurrence)

HERPES ZOSTER—Patients under 60 years of age (Note persistence and recurrence. Also note any Herpes Simplex—location, persistence and recurrence; if anal infection, note disability factors)

FEVER—Three months or more. Chart reading over period observed. You may have the patient keep a home record.

DIARRHEA—Three months or more. (Note frequency, times of day, patient's need for access to toilet facilities)

EMACIATION—Weight loss of 10% or more of body weight or 15 or more pounds. Chart weight records over period observed.

CENTRAL OR PERIPHERAL NEUROLOGIC DEFICIT (If applicable, relate to any factors of dementia)

PNEUMONIA (State type, duration, and necessity of hospitalization with course of treatment)

Minor

NIGHT SWEATS—Three months or more in duration (Note effect on continuous night rest)

FATIGUE (Note degree, progression over period observed, frequency of rest required, effect on patient's ability to function in work-related or personal capacities)

PRURITUS—One month or more duration (Location, frequency, noticeable scratching by patient)

BULLOUS IMPETIGO (Severity, location(s), recurrence, duration, frequency, effect on patient's physical appearance and grooming)

REFRACTORY DERMATOPHYTOSIS (Severity, location(s), recurrence, duration, frequency, effect on patient's physical appearance and grooming)

EXTENSIVE MOLLUSCUM CONTAGIOSUM (Severity, location(s), recurrence, duration, frequency, effect on patient's physical appearance and grooming)

EXTENSIVE SEBORRHEIC DERMATITIS & ECZEMA (Severity, location(s), recurrence, duration, frequency, effect on patient's physical appearance and grooming)

PERSISTENT SINUSITIS (Severity, frequency, associated headaches, post nasal drip, runny nose)

NAUSEA, MALAISE, DYSPNEA, AND HEADACHES (Please note these if observed and how they may be associated with patient's disease and ability to function)

Laboratory

Attach all reports to evaluation.

HTLV–III Antibody Positive

HTLV–III Virus Culture Positive

Leukopenia—White blood count of less than 4,000/mm³

Anemia—Hematocrit 35 or less

Thrombocytopenia—Platelet count of less than 100,000/mm³

Serum Globulins—3.5 grams/dl or more

Sedimentation Rate—20 or more

Serum cholesterol—Less than 135 mg

Immunologic

Attach all reports to evaluation.

Helper T-cell Count—Under 400/mm³

Helper/Suppressive ratio of less than 1.0

Cutaneous anergy—Negative to 3 or more skin tests

Karnofsky Performance Status Scale

(Circle)

100	Normal, no complaints, no evidence of disease
90	Able to carry on normal activity, minor signs of symptoms of disease
80	Normal activity with effort, some signs and symptoms of disease
70	Cares for self, unable to carry on normal activity or do normal work
60	Requires occasional assistance, able to care for most of his/her needs
50	Requires considerable assistance and frequent medical care
40	Disabled, requires special care and assistance
30	Severely disabled, hospitalization is indicated although death not imminent
20	Hospitalization necessary, very sick, action support treatment necessary
10	Moribund, fatal processes progressing rapidly
0	Dead

List of Medications (including dosage, instructions for taking)

Additional Comments and Observations

Disability is expected to last _____ months.

Disability is expected to result in death.　　Yes　　No

　　　　　　　　　　　　　　　　　　　　　(Circle one)

Name of Reporting Physician　　　　　　　　Title

Address　　　　　　　　　　　　　　　　　Phone

City and State　　　　Zip Code　　　　　　Best time to call if
　　　　　　　　　　　　　　　　　　　　　necessary

Signature　　　　　　　　　　　　　　　　Date

ARC Disability for Social Security Benefits: Mental Evaluation Instructions

The following evaluation form covers most aspects of mental disorders experienced by patients suffering from AIDS-Related Complex (ARC). The form also provides information normally used to develop Social Security claims involving mental disorders.

The form may be used as a guide to prepare a narrative report which may be substituted. ARC patient claims are assessed on a case-by-case basis by Social Security. *It is important to stress how each finding is related to the patient's disability, ability to perform Substantial Gainful Activity (SGA, any type of work), and daily personal activities.* A statement of findings alone may not suffice to meet SSA Disability listings.

The symptoms and findings should indicate any variance observed over time. The severity of mental impairment should be stated and, if applicable, assessment of the Mental Residual Functional Capacity (RFC) (that is, concentration, orientation, interaction with others, memory, etc.). Medical impairment(s) will be developed by the patient's treating physician via another pertinent format. However, if physical impairments related to the ARC patient's mental or neurological condition are observed, they should be noted.

Dementia and emaciation (wasting disorder) have been added as two disorders utilized to confirm an AIDS diagnosis by the federal Centers for Disease Control. The Social Security Administration adopted these findings as indicative of AIDS for the purpose of Presumptive Disability effective 09/01/87. There is no anticipated expansion or variation from the previous SSA disability criteria for dementia or emaciation (wasting disorder—loss of 10% or more of body weight or 15 or more pounds). These disorders should be fully developed for ARC patients.

The majority of ARC patient findings include severe diarrhea and fatigue. It is important to show the *severity* and *frequency* of these disorders (e.g., "needs immediate and continuous access to toilet facilities due to diarrhea"; "bed rest and frequent naps are required throughout the day due to fatigue"). It would be helpful to relate how these particular findings would preclude normal work activity.

For Social Security purposes, disability must be expected to last at least 12 months. A statement should be included in your report regarding the length of time the disability is expected to last.

The form may be placed in the patient's file and annotated and updated each examination or office visit. It is important to state how the mental findings disable the patient under each applicable category.

A comprehensive narrative report for Social Security purposes should include the following:

- Medical history
- Longitudinal history
- Findings
- Disabling factors of mental disorder(s)
- Any neurologic deficits noted
- Patient's ability to perform any type of work as a result of his/her mental condition
- Residual functional capacity (if any) (that is, concentration, orientation, time and place, interaction with others, memory, etc.)
- Physical disabilities observed
- Prognosis
- Length of time disability is expected to last

Sample Mental Health Narrative

_____ entered treatment with me on March 28, 1988 for anxiety and depression due to his ARC. Thus far we have had seven sessions. When _____ entered treatment he supported himself by working full time. During the course of our work together it became apparent that due to the physical and emotional impact of the ARC, _____ could no longer work without severe emotional consequences. It appeared that the emotional stress impacted _____'s health. He became easily fatigued and had frequent bouts with illness. His experience of job-related stress increased as he became more emotionally and physically incapable of continuing adequate job performance. Due to the stress and considerable emotional pain _____ was experiencing, I assessed him as being at high risk for a relapse into an addictive pattern of substance abuse from which _____ was three years abstinent.

_____ resigned his position, which reduced his stress considerably. In addition, this freed up his time, giving him the opportunity for visits to the clinic so his health could be monitored and treated. It afforded him time to get much-needed rest as well as giving him the time to attend support groups.

In my judgment as a mental health professional, _____ is emotionally incapable of working for at least 18 months, probably indefinitely. This is attributable to the anxiety and depression he experiences due to the ARC. Although I am not qualified as a medical doctor to assess _____'s physical health, it is apparent that his fatigue and frequent bouts with illness, in addition to his need for much rest and frequent visits to the clinic, compound his disability. A further concern and consideration for disability is _____'s fifteen-year history of drug addiction, including IV drugs. _____ is now three years abstinent and involved in Narcotics Anonymous. Returning to work, which would compound _____'s stress, is contraindicated as it would put him at high risk for a relapse into active drug addiction.

I used the DSM–III diagnostic codes. I diagnosed _____ with an adjustment disorder with mixed emotional features, 309.28. In addition, 304.73, which is dependence on a combination of opioid and other nonalcoholic substances in remission and 303.93, alcohol dependence in remission.

If you have any questions, my phone number is _____.

Dictated by _____.

Evaluation Form for Mental Disorders

(Generic, nongovernment form to be submitted along with SSA's own forms to increase chance of being found "disabled"—especially useful in "ARC-only" cases.)

Patient Name

Social Security Number

Date Patient First Examined

Date of Most Recent Examination

Frequency of Visits

Onset Date of Disability
(This should not be today's date, or the date the patient first sought care from you or another practitioner, or even the date the patient first fully accepted the reality of his symptoms. Rather it is your best medical judgment as to the date—perhaps well in the past—when his disease first began preventing effective, ongoing work ability.)

A narrative report, covering the following points, may be substituted instead of this form.

Note: The evidence needed to evaluate this patient's disability claim must be as objective and as specific as possible. Specific examples of the patient's behavior, thinking, and functioning are necessary to make a determination. Verbatim quotations of the patient's speech are frequently useful.

1. GENERAL OBSERVATIONS: Does the patient require assistance to keep his/her appointments? In what way and by whom? Please describe posture, gait, mannerisms, and general appearance.

2. GENERAL ILLNESS: What are the patient's complaints and symptoms? How and when did they begin? Does the patient describe complaints (Verbatim quotes)?

3. PAST HISTORY OF MENTAL DISORDER: Inpatient and outpatient, dates, location, and courses of treatment.

4. FAMILY, SOCIAL, AND ENVIRONMENTAL HISTORY: Family, education, marriage, divorce, work, sickness, alcohol, drug abuse, prison, etc.

5. MENTAL STATUS EXAMINATION: For each of the items listed below, please record enough detailed observations to recreate the patient's clinical picture.

A. Attitude and Behavior: Please describe the patient's general attitude, e.g., pleasant, hostile, relaxed, fearful, etc., and any examples of noteworthy behaviors, such as tearfulness, motor activity, emotional liability, etc.

B. Intellectual Functioning/Sensorium: Please describe and provide specific examples of orientation, memory, concentration, perceptual or thinking disturbance, judgment, etc. If intellectual functioning or organic involvements have been measured with standardized tests, please include any available results, including date of testing, and please attach test results to this report.

C. Affective Status: Please present any evidence of anxiety, depression, phobias, manic syndrome, inappropriate affect, somatoform disorder, suicidal/homicidal ideation, etc. Please describe objective signs of any diagnosed affective disorder, such as weight change, insomnia, decreased energy, feelings of guilt or worthlessness, anhedonia, etc.

D. Reality Contact: Does the patient present delusions, hallucinations, paranoid ideation, confusion, mood swings, emotional liability, emotional withdrawal and/or isolation, catatonic or grossly disorganized behavior, loosening of associations, etc.? Please describe in detail.

6. CURRENT LEVEL OF FUNCTIONING: Indicate to what extent (if any) the patient's current mental condition interferes with each of the following *with supporting data and examples.*

A. Present Daily Activities: Discuss the degree of assistance or direction needed to properly care for personal affairs, do shopping, cook, use public transportation, pay bills, maintain residence, care for grooming and hygiene, etc. In what ways, if any, have the patient's daily activities changed as a result of the patient's mental condition?

B. Social Functioning: Describe the patient's capacity to interact appropriately and communicate effectively with family members, neighbors, friends, landlords, fellow employees, etc. In what ways, if any, have these changed as a result of the patient's condition?

C. Concentration and Task Completion: Describe the patient's ability to sustain focused attention, complete everyday household routines, follow and understand simple written or oral instructions, etc. In what ways, if any, have these changed as a result of the patient's condition?

D. Adaptation to Work or Work-like Situations: Describe the patient's ability to adapt to stresses common to the work environment, including decision-making, attendance, schedules, and interaction with supervisors. In what ways, if any, have these changed as a result of the patient's condition?

7. CURRENT MEDICATIONS (if any): List dosage and response.

8. DIAGNOSIS: (DSM–III)

9. PROGNOSIS: Can the patient's condition be expected to improve? If so, when do you consider significant change likely to occur?

10. COMPETENCY: Is patient competent to manage funds on his/her own behalf:
_____Yes   _____No

11. ADDITIONAL COMMENTS: Attach additional pages, if necessary.

Disability is expected to last _____ months.
Disability is expected to result in death.   Yes   No
                                             (Circle one)

Name of Reporting Practitioner	Title

Address	Phone

City and State Zip Code	Best time to call if necessary

Signature	Date

Claimant/Physician Functional Capacity Report

(Generic, nongovernment form to be submitted along with SSA's own forms to increase chance of being found "disabled"—especially useful in "ARC-only" cases.)

Instructions

Please complete the attached form, indicating the degree of functioning and categories that most accurately describe your ARC condition on a daily basis.

Name _____

Address _____

SSN _____

Telephone No. _____

ONSET DATE OF DISABILITY _____

(This should not be today's date, or the date you first sought medical care, or even the date you first fully accepted the reality of your symptoms. Rather it is your best judgment as to the date—perhaps well in the past—when your disease first began preventing effective, ongoing work ability. Do not exaggerate how long you have remained able to work for reasons of self-esteem, pride, or shame—this could result in inaccurate information which might limit your benefits.)

Please check appropriate box and indicate number(s) where requested.

Fatigue

I require rest or nap(s) (Check box and indicate # where appropriate)

1. Only get out of bed for medical appointments, etc. _____
2. Twice or more per day _____ # of hours _____
3. Once a day _____ # of hours _____
4. Rarely require naps or rests _____
5. I suffer ramifications of medication(s), anemia from AZT, weakness, etc.

   yes _____   no _____

Diarrhea

I experience diarrhea: (Check box and indicate # where appropriate)

Daily _____   Frequently _____

Occasionally _____   Never _____

I normally experience diarrhea:

A.M. hours _____   # of stools _____

P.M. hours _____   # of stools _____

I am incontinent: (Please circle)

Frequently   Occasionally   Never

Night Sweats and Fevers

I experience night sweats: (Please circle)

Nightly   Frequently   Occasionally   Never

I experience fevers: (Please circle)

A.M. hours _____   P.M. hours _____   Both A.M. & P.M. _____

I experience fevers:

Daily   Frequently   Occasionally   Never

Average fever temperature _____°

Night Rest

My night rest is interrupted: (Please circle)

Nightly   Frequently   Occasionally   Never

My night rest is interrupted by: (Please check any and all appropriate categories)

Night sweats _____

Fevers _____

Headaches _____

Diarrhea _____

Respiratory problems _____

Sinusitis _____

Nausea _____

Itching or pain caused by herpes or other skin condition _____

Anxiety, nervousness, depression _____

I take sleeping medication: Yes _____   No _____

Mobility

I take walks: (Please circle)

Daily   Frequently   Occasionally   Never

I groom myself:

Daily   Frequently   Occasionally   Never

I require assistance to groom myself: Yes _____   No _____

I require rest during grooming: Yes _____   No _____

I clean my apartment, do my own laundry, etc.:

Daily   Weekly   Monthly   Never

I require assistance with household chores: Yes _____   No _____

When I go out I utilize:

A car _____   Public transportation _____   Taxi _____

Someone drives me _____

I go out of my home to visit friends or relatives:

Frequently   Occasionally   Never

(Please check appropriate box)

Prepare my own meals   _____

Cook pre-prepared or canned foods   _____

Meal delivery program   _____

Friends assist with cooking   _____

Mental Disposition

I experience:

Depression   Anxiety   Confusion   Anger

Fear   No Mental Problems

Alcohol Abuse   Drug Abuse

Alcoholism   Drug Addiction

The above circled categories regulate my mental ability and significantly impair or prevent my daily functioning:

Daily   Frequently   Occasionally   Never

I have difficulty with my memory, concentration, orientation:

Yes _____   No _____

I think of suicide: Yes _____   No _____

Respiratory Functioning (Please circle)

I suffer from respiratory problems:

Constantly   Frequently   Occasionally   Never

I have shortness of breath:

Daily   Nightly   Frequently   Occasionally   Never

I have shortness of breath on exertion:

Frequently   Occasionally   Never

I cough:

Frequently   Occasionally   Never

I choke from coughing:

Frequently   Occasionally   Never

I have had bouts of pneumonia (non-PCP):

Frequently   Occasionally   Never

Flexibility/Stamina (Please circle)

I can walk for   0   1   2   3   4   5   6   7   8   hours

I can stand for   0   1   2   3   4   5   6   7   8   hours

I can sit for   0   1   2   3   4   5   6   7   8   hours

I can bend: Frequently   Occasionally   Never

I can lift: 10 lbs.   20 lbs.   30 lbs.   40 lbs.   50 lbs.

I can lift the above-indicated weight:

Frequently   Occasionally   Never

I can reach: Frequently   Occasionally   Never

Other

List other conditions that are not listed that may affect you in your daily functioning (neuropathy, lymph infections, etc.)

I expect my disability to last _____ months.

I expect my disability to result in death.   Yes   No

                                                (Circle one)

The levels of Residual Functional Capacity indicated by this patient are an accurate description of his/her abilities and are consistent with the HIV symptoms diagnosed.

Patient Signature _____

Physician Signature _____

Physician Name_____

Title _____

Address _____

_____

Telephone No. _____

Daily Activities Questionnaire

(THIRD PARTY INFORMATION)

Applicant Name

IDENTITY OF CONTACT

Name   Relationship

Address   Number   Street   City   Zip Code   Telephone Number

How long have you known the applicant? How frequently do you see the applicant?

To the extent of your personal knowledge and direct observation of the applicant, please answer the following questions about his/her daily activities and social functioning. We are especially interested in whether there has been a change in the applicant's behavior since the onset of his/her condition.

Please comment on the applicant's ability to initiate and complete activities or tasks in an appropriate manner and the amount of assistance, if any, that the applicant requires to do so.

GENERAL INFORMATION

1. Where does the applicant currently live?

    _____ Home _____ Apartment _____ Boarding House _____ Nursing Home
    _____ Other

If other, please explain.

2. With whom does the applicant live?

_____ Alone _____ With Family _____ With Friends _____ Board and Care
_____ Other

If other, please explain.

ACTIVITIES OF DAILY LIVING

1. How does the applicant generally spend a typical day?

---

2. A. What are the applicant's normal sleeping hours?

B. What difficulties, if any, does the applicant have sleeping?

---

3. A. What difficulties does the applicant have caring for his/her personal needs (e.g., grooming, dressing, cleaning, etc.)? Does the applicant require any type of assistance? If yes, please explain.

B. Have the applicant's grooming habits changed since he/she became ill? If yes, please explain.

---

4. A. Who prepares and cooks the applicant's meals?

B. What type of foods does the applicant cook? How often?

C. Does anyone help the applicant prepare his/her meals? If yes, how much do they help the applicant?

5. A. What shopping does the applicant do? How frequently? Does anyone have to help the applicant with shopping?

   B. Who pays the applicant's bills and manages his/her checking and/or savings accounts? If someone helps the applicant, please explain.

6. A. What household chores does the applicant do (i.e., cleaning, maintenance, laundry, ironing, etc.)?

   B. Does the applicant need any help completing these chores? If so, please explain.

7. A. How often does the applicant go outside the home?

   B. What assistance, if any, does the applicant need to get out?

   C. Does the applicant have a driver's license and drive a car?   _____ Yes
                                                                       _____ No

   D. Does the applicant use public transportation?   _____ Yes   _____ No

8. What type of recreational activities or hobbies does the applicant enjoy and spend time on?

9. How much does the applicant listen to the radio or watch TV? What types of programs does he/she listen to or watch? Is the applicant able to remember the programs that he/she heard or watched?

10. How much does the applicant read? What does he/she read (e.g., books, newspapers, magazines)? Is the applicant able to remember what he/she read?

SOCIAL FUNCTIONING

1. What difficulties, if any, does the applicant have getting along with family, friends, co-workers or others? Please explain.

2. How often does the applicant visit family and friends, or have them visit him/her?

3. Is anyone dependent upon the applicant for care (e.g., spouse, children, parents, pets)? If so, what assistance does the applicant provide?

4. What community, church, sports, or social groups does the applicant belong to? Is he/she active in these groups? How does the applicant participate?

5. How often does the applicant attend movies, concerts, or other entertainment activities? Does he/she go alone or with others?

6. How have the applicant's social activities changed since his/her condition began?

PERSONAL INFORMATION

1. Does the applicant ever have problems concentrating or remembering? If so, please give examples.

2. When the applicant begins a task or chore does he/she ever have trouble following instructions or finishing the job? If so, please give examples.

3. Does the applicant exhibit any unusual behaviors or fears? Please explain.

4. Please comment on any additional factors or observations that you feel will be helpful to us in reaching a decision about the applicant's disability claim.

Coping with the Social Security Disability Determination Process

Probably the most difficult, mysterious, and frustrating task PWAs and their advocates face involves disability determination for SSDI and SSI. Not only are the medical disability standards unclear to most of the interested public—so are the methods of evaluation, the kinds of medical data to be reviewed, the stages and processes for claim consideration, and even the exact organizations handling the various parts of the process. This appendix briefly addresses these issues and offers some guidance for successful management of SSDI and SSI disability claims.

SSDI/SSI Disability Standards

The Social Security Act defines disability as "the inability to engage in any substantial gainful activity by reason of any medically determinable physical or mental impairment which can be expected to result in death or which has lasted or can be expected to last for a continuous period of not less than 12 months." Substantial gainful activity (SGA) is the ability to earn at least $300 monthly in any activity or occupation which exists in the national economy of the United States.

How does Social Security determine what illnesses, injuries or conditions—and of what severity and under what circumstances—constitute an inability to engage in SGA? It does this via detailed regulations set forth at 20 C.F.R. Parts 404 and 416. The first, more definitive method is by setting forth a *Listing of Impairments* (contained in appendices to Parts 404 and 416), which not only contains the 100 or so most common disabling illnesses, injuries, and conditions, but also sets forth the "proof" standards for evaluating claims which allege these impairments—diagnoses, prognoses, symptoms, and laboratory, X-ray and serological tests, etc.

To oversimplify somewhat, an impairment or combination of impairments will "meet" a listing section if it (they) presents the specific symptoms and "proofs" listed for that (those) impairment(s). In addition, an impairment (or combination of impairments) can sometimes "equal" a listing even if it does not "meet" one: it does this when a patient's symptoms and "proofs" are at least equivalent in severity to those called for in a listed impairment. This can happen where (a) the impairment is listed, but the patient does not present all the called-for "proofs," but does have *other* proofs, at least as strong, which support the impairment diagnosis; (b) the impairment isn't listed, but a closely related or parallel impairment is, and the patient's "proofs" meet the standards for *that* impairment; or (c) the patient has several impairments, the "proofs" of which do not individually meet listings rules, but which *together* are equivalent to standards for a closely related listing's "proofs."

Where an impairment, or set of impairments, does not "meet" or "equal" the criteria of the *Listing of Impairments,* Social Security evaluates medical proofs of an applicant's "Residual Functional Capacity" (RFC). This is a medical assessment of a person's work setting abilities in spite of functional limitations and environmental restrictions imposed by medically determinable impairments; in other words, it is an evaluation of the capacity for sustained performance of physical and mental job requirements. In short, the RFC method amounts to a sort of individually tailored disability determination for those whose "square peg" conditions cannot fit into the "round holes" of the *Listing.* Complementing and elaborating on the RFC method, SSA has issued detailed standards to consider the educational levels, vocational experiences, and ages of applicants in conjunction with medical data. These rules—most notably the highly complex "grids" which jointly "weigh" medical, educational, vocational, and age factors in the disability determination "scales"—essentially say that the less educated one is, the more unskilled/"hard labor" one's vocational experience was, and/or the older one is, then the more likely one is to be found disabled with a "doubtful" or "borderline" impairment.

What all of this means, one may well conclude, is that "full-blown AIDS" ought to qualify for, and appear in, the *Listing of Impairments,* while ARC is to be considered via the RFC/educational/vocational/age "individualized" method. And, in fact, this is more or less true: while, by late 1989, SSA had not codified AIDS into its *Listing of Impairments* in 20 C.F.R., it *did* issue regulations (see D–1c) accepting AIDS for SSI "presumptive disability" purposes and published criteria similar to the *Listing of Impairments* for AIDS in the *Program Operating Manual System* (POMS) used by its field claims representatives (see D–1a); and ARC continues to be considered under the RFC method (see SSA issuance at D–1b).

Applying SSDI/SSI Disability Standards: The Role of the DDS

SSA asks SSDI/SSI claimants to complete not only SSDI and SSI application forms, but also an 8-page *Disability Report,* a 6-page *Vocational Report,* and several supplementary forms. In addition, applicants must submit—or authorize SSA to send for—the medical practitioner's narrative report as well as copies of all physician, clinic, and hospital records. SSA arranges for the evaluation of the disability-related material by what is called the Disability Determination Service (DDS)—an arm of the state vocational rehabilitation agency working under SSA contract. Where all necessary narrative reports and coherent medical records have not been submitted by the applicant or his advocate along with the SSDI/SSI application (which, unfortunately, is almost always the case), the overworked and paperwork-overwhelmed DDS attempts to collect them from doctors and hospitals. Doctors, their staffs, and hospital record departments are *themselves* not only overwhelmed by paperwork backlogs—they rarely know what quality, coherency, or persuasiveness in narrative forms or records the DDS needs to make a finding of disability. As a practical matter, it's easier for a DDS evaluator (frustrated with an inadequately documented, overdue case file) to deny a claim for medical insufficiency than to coax useful, pertinent data from backlogged and unresponsive doctors and medical records staffs.

The result is that only about one-third of SSDI applicants are initially found eligible, and even upon reconsideration, only about one-sixth win awards. Yet at the next stage of the SSA eligibility process—Administrative Law Judge (ALJ) hearings—more than half win eligibility. The reason for this discrepancy is not hard to find: applicants and advocates who carelessly assembled their medical records and doctors' reports (or who even fail to do so at all, leaving assembly to the vagaries of DDS/medical records staff interaction), are shocked into reality by initial and reconsideration denials—they seek expert advice from poverty law programs or privately paid disability law attorneys. These advocates review the inadequate, unresponsive, and poorly written submissions which brought about the denials, and then do what should have been done in the first place—they *themselves* gather medical records (hand-carried, not by mailed requests) and procure adequate doctors' narrative reports (if necessary, they demand that they be rewritten) and responses to impairment-specific, tailored questionnaires.

Tips for Handling SSDI/SSI Claims for PWAs and PWARCs

• Gather by hand medical records from clinics and hospitals—and submit them to SSA with the application (or if there are unavoidable delays, hand-deliver them to the DDS if the case file has already been forwarded there).

• Personally submit and then hand carry to SSA (or the DDS) the practitioner questionnaires printed in this appendix. Instructions precede each questionnaire.

• If possible (some doctors will simply not do so), have one's doctor and therapist draft narrative reports *as well*. Show them the samples and outline instructions in this appendix.

• Don't hesitate to reject, and point out the failings of, inadequate, skimpy, or lukewarm doctor reports—not only do doctors *hate* to write these, but they are often too self-confident to take helpful advice, and too upbeat in their diagnoses (in order to boost patient morale). Many—and, as the hearings reversals suggest, *most*—doctor reports prove to be woefully inadequate on the first try.

• Mention, and secure records and reports about, seemingly unrelated conditions, whether in the present or in the past.

• Don't be overly optimistic or unrealistic about your work or personal care abilities—this could result in a denial.

• Be especially careful to include statements from practitioners, applicants themselves, and those who know them about embarrassing, personal maladies, conditions and even habits. These might include: mental or emotional problems, treatments, therapy, or hospitalizations; alcohol or drug history or usage or addiction, including usage to cope with depression, anxiety, or discrimination; drug or alcohol detoxifications, and any recovery program attempts; incontinence, bed-wetting, or overly frequent diarrhea; workplace or social problems with appearance (such as dress, personal manner, KS lesions, or wasting); hostility, depression, paranoia; excessive medication-induced mood changes, coordination problems, or other side effects; and the psychological impact of anti-gay or anti-minority discrimination.

- Be sure to detail examples of social life, travel, shopping, cooking, housekeeping, grooming, recreational, sports, volunteer, religious, and relationship limitations caused by medical condition.

- Discuss pain, gait limitations, and sleep disruptions.

- Don't hesitate to submit written third party reports (see form in this appendix) from lovers, roommates, spouses, friends, bosses, coworkers, neighbors, clergymen or whoever else can support the application.

- File the SSDI and/or SSI application *in person* at the Social Security office (don't be talked into using the telephone or mail-in method!) with a *real, live claims representative*—and get his or her direct telephone number for follow-up. Mistakes on mailed-in forms become part of the permanent record; in-person applicants have on-the-spot help in answering questions and correcting mistakes.

- Ask the SSA claims representative for the name, address, and *telephone number* of the DDS worker or branch to which the claim will be sent for review.

- Those with "full-blown AIDS" applying for SSI as well as SSDI should always *insist* on an *immediate* "presumptive disability" determination.

- After a decent interval, call the DDS worker or branch and inquire what additional information, records, files, or statements you might submit (in addition to what they already have) to assist case processing.

- *Never* mail *your only copy* of any document, report, or form and *always* (if possible) hand deliver submissions to SSA or the DDS.

- *Always immediately request a reconsideration or hearing* when an application is denied.

- Needy PWAs and PWARCs with difficult or denied applications should contact the Neighborhood Legal Services or Legal Aid Society serving their area for free or low-cost help—their staffs are experts in the SSDI/SSI issues and procedures.

- PWAs and PWARCs who *do* have financial resources can secure referral to privately paid attorneys with disability expertise by telephoning the National Organization of Social Security Claimant Representatives, (800) 431–2804.

Remember, the best guarantees for a successful SSDI/SSI claim are hand-carried, well-documented, carefully written, and thorough physician narratives, questionnaires, and medical records which demonstrate how and in exactly what ways a patient's condition and symptoms prevent ongoing, sustained work activity.

Appendix E

Documents/Verifications Needed to Apply, by Program

Bring, if Applicable to Circumstances:	SSDI	SSI	AFDC	GA	EA	Food Stamps	VA	AZT/ Drugs	Medicaid	Hill-Burton & Hospital Programs	Housing	Energy Assistance
Pay stubs for prior 3 months and present month or note on earnings from employer		•	•	•	•	•	•	•	•	•	•	•
Green card/visa/passport/immigration/ naturalization papers	•	•	•	•	•	•	•	•	•	•	•	•
Bank account statements for last 3 months; IRAs; stock certificates		•	•	•	•	•	•	•	•	•	•	•
Letter from attending physician giving: detailed diagnosis and prognosis; results of supporting biopsies, and laboratory, serological, and X-ray tests; statement that patient cannot work for at least 1 year	•	•					•[1]					

Document	1	2	3	4	5	6	7	8	9	10	11
Doctor's disability statement on welfare medical exam form				●	●		●				
Copies of hospital/clinical medical records, which can be picked up by patient or someone with signed authorization at little or no cost											●
Life, health, and burial insurance policies, I.D. cards and booklets		●		●	●		●	●		●	●
Automobile title and registration	●			●	●		●	●		●	●
Marriage/divorce/separation/custody/child support papers (if seeking benefits also for spouse, ex-spouse, or children)				●	●	●[1]	●	●		●	●
Rent receipts/cancelled checks/leases/note from landlord	●	●		●	●		●	●		●	●
Military discharge (DD 214)	●	●		●	●	●				●	●
Utility bills	●	●		●	●		●	●		●	●
Deed, mortgage, or tax papers for own home	●	●		●	●		●	●		●	●

Bring, if Applicable to Circumstances	SSDI	SSI	AFDC	GA	EA	Food Stamps	VA	AZT/ Drugs	Medicaid	Hill-Burton & Hospital Programs	Housing	Energy Assistance
Birth certificate (not photocopy)	•	•	•	•	•	•	•	•	•		•	•
Note from employer on date applicant stopped "earning own way" as worker and began being paid only as a "disguised charity" by employer		•										
Driver's license or other picture I.D.	•	•	•	•	•	•	•	•	•	•	•	•
Social Security card for each applicant	•	•	•	•	•	•	•	•	•	•	•	•
Medical bills for prior 3 months and present month (if not received yet, pick up interim copies from hospital/doctor's office)		•				•	•	•	•	•	•	•
Note from doctor that applicant is home-bound and in need of aid-and-attendant services due to medical condition							•²		•²			
Copies of military hospital/clinic medical records							•³					

Children's birth certificates, school papers, and babysitting receipts (if living with children)

Voting registration (if registered)

List of jobs for past 15 years

Wage and tax forms (W-2's) for past 2 completed calendar years

All paystubs for current year or note from employer(s) describing earnings

Forms and papers on any other government or employer benefit program

Eviction/rent/mortgage/utility delinquency notes; police/fire reports on lost/stolen/damaged money or goods

Note from lover/roommate/landlord/relatives that applicant purchases/eats food separately

Bring, if Applicable to Circumstances:	SSDI	SSI	AFDC	GA	EA	Food Stamps	VA	AZT/ Drugs	Medicaid	Hill-Burton & Hospital Programs	Housing	Energy Assistance
Note from lover/roommate/landlord/relatives that applicant pays his share of household costs, or if he has no income now, is being "loaned" value of his share to be repaid out of future benefits	●		●[4]	●[4]		●[4]						
Proof of age or disability of sibling(s)/parent(s) if living with sibling(s)/parent(s) over age 60 or disabled	●[4]		●[4]	●[4]		●						

Source: Analysis of program rules and application forms by author.

Do *not* delay applying to gather documents/verifications; it could mean loss or delay in payments and benefits. Extra submission time is granted to all applicants.

[1] Only if applying for VA pension.

[2] If seeking extra VA payments as "housebound" or in need of "aid-and-attendant" care; or seeking home health aid/chore aid/personal care attendant/homemaker services from Medicaid or adult social services/Title XX.

[3] Only if seeking compensation payments from VA.

[4] Only if requested by program worker.

Appendix F

Regional Offices of HHS

Region I
(CT, ME, MA, NH, RI, VT)
Room 1211
JFK Federal Building
Boston, MA 02203
(617) 565–1322

Region II
(NJ, NY, PR, VI)
Room 3821
26 Federal Plaza
New York, NY 10278
(212) 264–1121

Region III
(DE, DC, MD, PA, VA, WV)
3535 Market Street
P.O. Box 7760
Philadelphia, PA 19101
(215) 596–6571

Region IV
(AL, FL, GA, KY, MS, NC, SC, TN)
Suite 523
101 Marietta Tower
Atlanta, GA 30323
(404) 331–2361

Region V
(IL, IN, MI, MN, OH, WI)
Suite 941
175 West Jackson Boulevard
Chicago, IL 60604
(312) 353–9804

Region VI
(AR, LA, NM, OK, TX)
Room 2335
1200 Main Tower Building
Dallas, TX 75202
(214) 767–6301

Region VII
(IA, KS, MO, NE)
Room 275
New Federal Office Building
601 East 12th Street
Kansas City, MO 64104
(816) 374–2408

Region VIII
(CO, MT, ND, SD, UT, WY)
Federal Building, Room 1194
1961 Stout Street
Denver, CO 80294
(303) 564–4721

Region IX
(AZ, CA, HI, NV)
14th Floor
100 Van Ness Avenue
San Francisco, CA 94102
(415) 556–8982

Region X
(AK, ID, OR, WA)
Mail Stop 409
2901 Third Avenue
Seattle, WA 98121
(206) 442–0511

Appendix G

National Advocacy/Resource Organizations

AIDS Action Council
2033 M Street, N.W.
Washington, DC 20036
(202) 293–2886

AIDS Benefits Counselors
1547 California Street
San Francisco, CA 94109
(415) 673–3780; (415) 227–5884

AIDS Legal Referral Panel
Bay Area Lawyers for Individual
   Freedom
Suite 400
1663 Mission Street
San Francisco, CA 94103
(415) 864–8186

American Association of Blood Banks
1117 North 19th Street
Arlington, VA 22209
(703) 528–8200

American Association of Physicians for
   Human Rights (AAPHR)
2940 16 Street, Room 309
San Francisco, CA 94103
(415) 558–9353

American Association of Retired
   Persons (AARP)
1909 K Street, N.W.
Washington, DC 20049
(202) 872–4700

American Foundation for AIDS
   Research (AmFAR)
5900 Wilshire Boulevard
2nd Floor–East Satellite
Los Angeles, CA 90036
(213) 857–5900
or
40 W. 57th St., Suite 406
New York, NY 10019
(212) 333–3118

American Hospital Association
50 F Street, N.W.
Washington, DC 20001
(202) 638–1100

American Medical Association (Health
   Policy Agenda)
535 North Dearborn Street
Chicago, IL 60610
(312) 645–5271; (800) 621–8335

American Public Health Association
1015 15th Street, N.W.
Washington, DC 20005
(202) 789–6500

Computerized AIDS Information
   Network (CAIN)
1213 North Highland Avenue
P.O. Box 38777
Hollywood, CA 90038
(213) 464–7400, ext. 277

Disabled American Veterans
807 Maine Avenue, S.W.
Washington, DC 20202
(202) 554–3501

Legal Counsel for the Elderly (LCE)
1133 20th Street, N.W.
Washington, DC 20036
(202) 662–4933

Mental Health Law Project
2021 L Street, N.W.
Washington, DC 20036
(202) 467–5730

Mothers of AIDS Patients (MAP)
P.O. Box 3132
San Diego, CA 92103
(619) 293–3985; (619) 576–6366

National AIDS Network (NAN)
2033 M Street, N.W.
Washington, DC 20036
(202) 293–2437

National Association of People With
  AIDS (NAPWA)
Suite 415
2025 Eye Street, N.W.
Washington, DC 20006
(202) 429–2856

National Association of Residential Care
  Facilities
Suite 209
1205 West Main Street
Richmond, VA 23220
(804) 355–3265

National Clearinghouse for Legal
  Services (Clearinghouse Review)
Suite 400
407 South Dearborn Street
Chicago, IL 60605
(312) 939–3830

National Coalition of Gay Sexually
  Transmitted Disease Services
P.O. Box 239
Milwaukee, WI 53201
(414) 277–7671

National Council of Churches AIDS
  Task Force
475 Riverside Dr., Room 572
New York, NY 10115
(212) 370–2421

National Council of Senior Citizens
925 15th Street, N.W.
Washington, DC 20005
(202) 347–8800

National Gay Rights Advocates
540 Castro Street
San Francisco, CA 94114
(415) 863–3624

National Health Care Campaign
1334 G Street, N.W.
Washington, DC 20005
(202) 639–8833

National Health Law Program
2639 South LaCienega Blvd.
Los Angeles, CA 90034
(213) 204–6010
or
2025 M Street, N.W.
Washington, DC 20036
(202) 887–5310

National Hemophilia Foundation
10104 Forest Avenue
Fairfax, VA 22030
(703) 352–2144

National Leadership Coalition on AIDS
Suite 202
1150 17th Street, N.W.
Washington, DC 20036
(202) 429–0930

National Senior Citizens Law Center
   (NSCLC)
1052 W. 6th St., 7th Floor
Los Angeles, CA 90017
(213) 482–3550
or
Suite 400
2025 M Street, N.W.
Washington, DC 20036
(202) 887–5280

Pension Rights Center
918 16th Street, N.W., Suite 704
Washington, DC 20006
(202) 296–3776

Vietnam Veterans of America
2001 S Street, N.W.
Washington, DC 20037
(202) 332–2700; (202) 797–8366
(800) 852–2369

Villers Foundation/Advocacy Associates
1334 G Street, N.W.
Washington, DC 20005
(202) 628–3030

State Level Advocacy/Resource Organizations, by State

Note: The American Association of Retired Persons (AARP) has a full-time staff at its headquarters who monitor developments and promote reforms in every state. They can be reached at the following address and telephone number (when writing, fill in the name of your state on the first line):

State Legislative Representative
American Association of Retired Persons (AARP)
1909 K Street, N.W.
Washington, DC 20049
(202) 662–4120

Alabama

Jefferson Clinic
Max Michael
1515 6th Avenue South
Birmingham, AL 35233
(205) 934–0159

Alabama Consortium of Legal Services
Marilyn S. Swears
207 Montgomery St., #500
Montgomery, AL 36104
(205) 264–1471

Commission on Aging
State Capitol
Montgomery, AL 36130
(205) 261–5743

Alaska

Alaska Legal Services Corporation
Robert K. Hickerson
550 W. 8th Ave., Suite 300
Anchorage, AK 99501
(907) 272–6282

Older Alaskans Commission
Pouch G, Mail Stop 0209
Juneau, AK 99811
(907) 465–3250

Arizona

Aging and Adult Administration
P.O. Box 6123
1400 West Washington St.
Phoenix, AZ 85005
(602) 255–4446

Arizona Statewide Legal Services
Cecilia D. Esquer
P.O. Box 311
Phoenix, AZ 85001
(602) 252–3432

Arizona Health Care Campaign
Phil Lopes
3131 E. 2nd Street
Tucson, AZ 85716
(602) 626–7946

Arkansas

Arkansas Legal Services
Tom McGowan
Suite 200, McFadden Building
615 West Markham Street
Little Rock, AR 72201
(501) 376–8015

Arkansas Senior Organizing Project
Scott Holladay
1408 Redsamen Park Road
Little Rock, AR 72202
(501) 661–1401

Arkansas State Office on Aging
Donaghey Bldg., Suite 1428
7th & Main Streets
Little Rock, AR 72201
(501) 371–2441

California

Legal Aid Foundation of Long Beach
Toby J. Rothschild
Security Pacific Bank Building
110 Pine Avenue, Suite 420
Long Beach, CA 90802
(213) 435–3501

Legal Aid Foundation of Los Angeles
Kathy Krause
1550 West 8th Street
Los Angeles, CA 90017
(213) 487–3320

Western Center on Law & Poverty
Mary Burdick
3535 West 6th Street
Los Angeles, CA 90020
(213) 487–7211

Department of Aging
1020 19th Street
Sacramento, CA 95814
(916) 322–5290

California Health Access Coalition
Maryann O'Sullivan
1535 Mission Street
San Francisco, CA 94103
(415) 431–7430

Campaign California
Cathy Calfo, director
1337 Santa Monica Mall, #301
Santa Monica, CA 90401
(213) 393–3701

Solano County Legal Assistance
David Monthiel
930 Marin Street
Vallejo, CA 94590
(707) 643–0054

Colorado

United Seniors of Colorado
Steven Moss
2021 Four Pikes Peak #5
Colorado Springs, CO 80904
(719) 471–8200

Aging and Adult Services Division
Department of Social Services
1575 Sherman St., Room 503
Denver, CO 80220
(303) 866–2586

Colorado Coalition of Legal Services
Daniel Taubman
1905 Sherman Street, #710
Denver, CO 80203
(303) 830–1551

Connecticut

Connecticut Citizen Action Group
Jeff Freiser, director
51 Van Dyke Avenue
Hartford, CT 06106
(203) 527–7191

Department on Aging
175 Main Street
Hartford, CT 06106
(203) 566–7725

Connecticut Citizen Action Group
Bob Reutenauer
33 Church Street
Willimantic, CT 06226
(203) 456–3157

New Haven Legal Assistance
Jon Alander
426 State Street
New Haven, CT 06510
(203) 777–4811

Delaware

Division of Aging
Department of Health and Social
  Services
1901 North Dupont Highway
New Castle, DE 19720
(302) 421–6791

District of Columbia

American Association of Retired
  Persons (AARP)
1909 K Street, N.W.
Washington, DC 20049
(202) 662–4120

Executive Director
Office on Aging
1424 K Street, N.W.
Washington, DC 20005
(202) 724–5622

Florida

Florida Legal Services
Scott Manion
345 So. Magnolia Dr., Suite A–27
Tallahassee, FL 32301
(904) 222–2151

Program Office of Aging and Adult
  Services
Department of Health and Rehabilitation
  Services
1323 Winewood Boulevard
Tallahassee, FL 32301
(904) 488–8922

Florida Consumers Federation
Frank Jackalone, director
937 Belvedere Road
West Palm Beach, FL 33405
(305) 832–6077

Georgia

Atlanta Legal Aid Society
Don Coleman
777 Cleveland Avenue, SW–202
Atlanta, GA 30315
(404) 761–5872

Georgia Legal Services Program
John L. Cromartie, Jr.
133 Luckie St., N.W., 8th Fl.
Atlanta, GA 30303
(404) 656–6021

Office of Aging
878 Peachtree St., N.E., Rm. 632
Atlanta, GA 30309
(404) 894–5333

Hawaii

Executive Office on Aging
1149 Bethel St., Room 307
Honolulu, HI 96813
(808) 548–2593

Idaho

Idaho Health Care Campaign
Gary Sandusky
688 North 9th
Boise, ID 83702
(208) 385–9146

Idaho Legal Aid Services
Ernesto G. Sanchez
P.O. Box 913
Boise, ID 83701
(208) 336–8980

Idaho Office on Aging
Room 114–Statehouse
Boise, ID 83720
(208) 334–3833

Idaho Fair Share
John Stocks, director
P.O. Box 1793
Coeur D'Alene, ID 83814
(208) 664–5518

Illinois

Illinois Council of Senior Citizens
Jan Schakowsky
1 Quincy Court, Ste. 114
Chicago, IL 60601
(312) 421–6262

Illinois Public Action Council
Robert Creamer, director
220 South State St., Rm. 714
Chicago, IL 60604
(312) 427–6262

Illinois State Support Center
Michael O'Connor
343 South Dearborn Street
Chicago, IL 60604
(312) 341–1070

Department on Aging
421 East Capitol Avenue

Springfield, IL 62706
(217) 785–3356

Indiana

Citizens' Action Coalition of Indiana
Chris Williams, director
3951 North Meridian
Indianapolis, IN 46208
(317) 921–1120

Indiana Department on Aging and
   Community Services
115 N. Pennsylvania St., Suite 1350
Indianapolis, IN 46204
(317) 232–7006

Indiana Health Care Campaign
John Cardwell
3951 N. Meridian, 3rd Fl.
Indianapolis, IN 46208
(317) 921–1120

Indiana Legal Services Support
Sandra Leek
107 North Pennsylvania, Ste. 1008
Indianapolis, IN 46204
(317) 631–1395

Iowa

Iowa Citizen Action Network
Mary Bergstrom
1st Ave & 3rd St., #210
Cedar Rapids, IA 52401
(319) 363–7208

Commission on Aging
914 Grand Ave., Suite 236
Des Moines, IA 50319
(515) 281–5187

Iowa Citizen Action Network
Ben Zachrich, director
424 10th St., #305
Des Moines, IA 50309
(515) 244–9311

Legal Services Corp. of Iowa, Inc.
Randy Youells
315 E. 5th Street, #709
Des Moines, IA 50309
(515) 243-2151

Kansas

Department of Aging
610 West 10th Street
Topeka, KS 66612
(913) 296-4986

Kansas Coalition on Aging
Mark Intermill
1195 Buchanan
Topeka, KS 66604
(913) 232-1456

Kentucky

Division for Aging Services
Department of Human Resources
DHR Building, 6th Floor
275 East Main Street
Frankfort, KY 40601
(502) 564-6930

Kentucky Legal Services Program
Anthony Martin
201 West Short Street
Lexington, KY 40507
(606) 233-3057

Louisiana

Office of Elderly Affairs
P.O. Box 80374
4528 Bennington Avenue
Baton Rouge, LA 70898-0374
(504) 925-1700

Louisiana Legal Consortium
Catherine LaFleur
1636 Toledano St., Ste. 305
New Orleans, LA 70115
(504) 891-6441

Maine

Bureau of Maine's Elderly
Department of Human Services
State House, Station No. 11
Augusta, ME 04333
(207) 289-2561

Maine People's Alliance
Mary Edgerton, director
P.O. Box 17534
Portland, ME 04101
(207) 761-4400

Pine Tree Legal Assistance
Pamela Anderson
P.O. Box 547, D.T.S.
Portland, ME 04112
(207) 774-4753

Maryland

Legal Aid Bureau, Inc.
Charles H. Dorsey, Jr.
714 East Pratt Street
Baltimore, MD 21202-3105
(301) 539-5340

Maryland Citizen Action Coalition
Janelle Cousino, director
2500 North Charles St.
Baltimore, MD 21218
(301) 235-5588

Office on Aging
State Office Building
301 West Preston Street
Baltimore, MD 21201
(301) 383-5064

Massachusetts

Department of Elder Affairs
38 Chauncy Street
Boston, MA 02111
(617) 727-7751

Massachusetts Fair Share
Cynthia Ward
20 East St., 6th Fl.
Boston, MA 02111–2803
(617) 654–9000

Massachusetts Health Action Alliance
Susan Sherry
25 West St., 2nd Floor
Boston, MA 02111
(617) 350–7279

Massachusetts Law Reform Institute
Allan G. Rodgers
69 Canal Street
Boston, MA 02114
(617) 742–9250

Michigan

Michigan Legal Services
Louis Lessem
220 Bagley Ave., #900
Detroit, MI 48226
(313) 964–4130

Michigan Health Care Campaign
Joe Tuchinsky
122 South Grand Ave., Suite 200
Lansing, MI 48933
(517) 372–7111

Offices of Services to the Aging
P.O. Box 30026
Lansing, MI 48909
(517) 373–8230

Minnesota

Minnesota Health Care Campaign
Kip Sullivan
324 Hennepin Ave., East
Minneapolis, MN 55414
(612) 379–7811

Minnesota Board on Aging
Metro Square Bldg., Room 204

7th and Roberts Streets
St. Paul, MN 55101
(612) 296–2544

Minnesota COACT
John Musick, director
2395 University Ave., Rm. 304
St. Paul, MN 55104
(612) 645–0115

Minnesota Legal Services Coalition
Charlie Singer
700 Minnesota Building
St. Paul, MN 55101
(612) 228–9105

Mississippi

Children's Defense Fund
Rims Barber
P.O. Box 1684
Jackson, MS 39205
(601) 355–7495

Legal Services Coalition
Louis Armstrong
P.O. Box 22887
Jackson, MS 39205
(601) 944–0765

Mississippi Council on Aging
Executive Building, Suite 301
Jackson, MS 39201
(601) 354–6590

Missouri

Division on Aging
Department of Social Services
Broadway State, P.O. Box 570
Jefferson City, MO 65101
(314) 751–3082

Missouri Citizen Labor Coalition
Tom Bixby, director
317 West 39th Terrace
Kansas City, MO 64111
(816) 531–2443

Montana

Community Services Division
P.O. Box 4210
Helena, MT 59604
(406) 444–3865

Montana Legal Services
Neil Haight
801 N. Last Chance Gulch
Helena, MT 59601
(406) 442–9830

Montana Senior Citizens' Association
Dorothy Bompart
616 Helena Ave., #300
Helena, MT 59624
(406) 443–5341

Nebraska

Department on Aging
P.O. Box 95044
301 Centennial Mall South
Lincoln, NE 68509
(402) 471–2306

Nevada

Division for Aging Services
Department of Human Resources
505 East King St., Room 101
Carson City, NV 89710
(702) 885–4210

Nevada Legal Services
Wayne Pressel
111 West Telegraph, Suite 101
Carson City, NV 89701
(702) 885–5110

New Hampshire

Council on Aging
14 Depot St.
Concord, NH 03301
(603) 271–2751

New Hampshire Citizen Action
Kate McGovern/Chrisinda Lynch,
    Co-directors
8 North Main Street
Concord, NH 03301
(603) 225–2097

New Hampshire Legal Assistance
Robert D. Gross
15 Green Street
Concord, NH 03301
(603) 225–4700

New Jersey

New Jersey Health Care Coalition
Al Evanoff
50 Corona Road
East Brunswick, NJ 08816
(201) 545–7520

New Jersey Citizen Action
Phyllis Salowe-Kaye, director
400 Main Street
Hackensack, NJ 07601
(201) 488–2804

Legal Services of New Jersey, Inc.
Melville D. Miller, Jr.
78 New Street
New Brunswick, NJ 08901
(201) 246–0770

Division on Aging
Department of Community Affairs
363 West State St., CN 807
Trenton, NJ 08625–0807
(609) 292–4833

New Mexico

New Mexico Legal Services Support
    Project
John Vail
109 Elm, S.E.
Albuquerque, NM 87102
(505) 243–6282

State Agency on Aging
224 East Palace Avenue, 4th Fl.
La Villa Rivera Building
Santa Fe, NM 87501
(505) 827–7640

New York

Citizen Action of New York
Karen Scharff, co-director
314 Central Avenue, #202
Albany, NY 12206
(518) 465–4600
or
Alan Charney, co-director
15 East Dutch St., #300
New York, NY 10038
(212) 962–0855

New York Health Care Campaign
Richard Kirsch
314 Central Avenue, #204
Albany, NY 12206
(518) 465–4600

Office for the Aging
New York State Executive Department
Empire State Plaza, Agency Bldg. No. 2
Albany, NY 12223
(518) 474–5731

Community Action For Legal Services,
    Inc.
Wilhelm Joseph
335 Broadway
New York, NY 10013
(212) 431–7200

Greater Upstate Law Project
Steven L. Brown
87 Clinton Avenue North
Rochester, NY 14604
(716) 454–6500

North Carolina

Division of Aging
708 Hillsboro St., Suite 200
Raleigh, NC 27603
(919) 733–3983

North Carolina Fair Share
Elisa Wolper, director
P.O. Box 12543
Raleigh, NC 27605
(919) 832–7130

North Carolina Legal Services Resource
    Center
Don Saunders
P.O. Box 27343
Raleigh, NC 27611
(919) 821–0042

North Dakota

Aging Services
Department of Human Services
State Capitol Building
Bismarck, ND 58505
(701) 224–2577

Legal Assistance of North Dakota
Pam Bartholomew
222 West Bowen Ave.
Bismarck, ND 58501
(701) 222–2110

Ohio

Ohio Public Interest Campaign
Ira Arlook, director
Burgess Bldg., 2nd Fl.
1406 West 6th St.
Cleveland, OH 44113
(216) 861–5200

Ohio Department of Aging
50 West Broad Street, 9th Fl.
Columbus, OH 43215
(614) 466-5500

Ohio Public Interest Campaign
Pete MacDowell
691 North High St., 2nd Fl.
Columbus, OH 43215
(614) 224-4111

Ohio State Legal Services
Tom Weeks
861 North High Street
Columbus, OH 43215
(614) 299-2114

Oklahoma

Oklahoma Health Care Project
Angela Monson
1504 South Walker
Oklahoma City, OK 73109
(405) 236-1911

Oklahoma Legal Services Center
Maggie Dover
110 Cameron Building
2901 Classen Boulevard
Oklahoma City, OK 73110
(405) 557-0020

Special Unit on Aging
Department of Human Services
P.O. Box 25352
Oklahoma City, OK 73125
(405) 521-2281

Oregon

Legal Aid Service
Louis Savage
900 Board of Trade Bldg.
310 S.W. 4th Avenue
Portland, OR 97204
(503) 224-4086

Oregon Fair Share
Bill Weissman, director
2111 East Burnside
Portland, OR 97214
(503) 239-7611

Oregon Health Action Campaign
Ellen Pinney
P.O. Box 12644
Portland, OR 97309
(503) 581-6830

Oregon Senior Services Division
313 Public Service Building
Salem, OR 97310
(503) 378-4728

Pennsylvania

Department of Aging
231 State Street, Room 307
Harrisburg, PA 17120
(717) 783-1550

Law Coordination Center
Laurence M. Lavin
118 Locust Street
Harrisburg, PA 17101
(717) 232-2602

Pennsylvania Legal Services Center
Howard Thorkelson
130 Walnut Street
Harrisburg, PA 17101
(717) 236-9486

Pennsylvania Public Interest Campaign
Tom Gluck
933 Rose Street
Harrisburg, PA 17102
(717) 232-2126

Pennsylvania Public Interest Coalition
Jeff Blum, director
1207 Chestnut, 4th Fl.
Philadelphia, PA 19107
(215) 568-8145

Rhode Island

Community Labor Coalition
1468 Broad Street
Providence, RI 02905
(401) 461–8200

Department of Elderly Affairs
79 Washington Street
Providence, RI 02903
(401) 277–2858

Rhode Island Health Care Campaign
Karen Akers
1468 Broad Street
Providence, RI 02905
(401) 941–7750

Rhode Island Legal Services
John Mola
77 Dorrance Street
Providence, RI 02903
(401) 274–2652

South Carolina

Commission on Aging
915 Main Street
Columbia, SC 29201
(803) 758–2576

South Carolina Fair Share
John Ruoff, Director
P.O. Box 8888
Columbia, SC 29202
(803) 345–5057

South Carolina Legal Services
Nancy McCormick
P.O. Box 7187
Columbia, SC 29202
(803) 252–0034

South Dakota

Office of Adult Services and Aging
Department of Social Services

Richard F. Kneip Building
700 North Illinois Street
Pierre, SD 57501–2291
(605) 773–3656

Tennessee

Commission on Aging
703 Tennessee Building
535 Church Street
Nashville, TN 37219
(615) 741–2056

Tennessee Association Legal Services
Stewart Clifton
833 Stahlman Building
211 Union Street
Nashville, TN 37201–1586
(615) 242–0438

Tennessee Health Care Campaign
Bert Perkey
205 Reidhurst Ave., #N204
Nashville, TN 37203
(615) 329–3720

Texas

Texas Alliance for Human Needs
Rosie Torres
2520 Longview
Austin, TX 78705
(512) 474–5019

Texas Department on Aging
210 Barton Springs Rd., 5th Fl.
Austin, TX 78704
(512) 475–2717

Texas Legal Services Center
Randall Chapman
210 Barton Springs Rd., #300
Austin, TX 78704
(512) 477–4562

Utah

Division of Aging and Adult Services
Department of Social Services
150 West North Temple, Box 2500
Salt Lake City, UT 84110–2500
(801) 533–6422

Utah Legal Services
Ann Milne
124 South 400 East, 4th Fl.
Salt Lake City, UT 84111
(801) 328–8891

Vermont

Vermont Legal Aid, Inc.
John Shullenberger
P.O. Box 1367
Burlington, VT 05402
(802) 863–2871

Office on Aging
103 South Main Street
Waterbury, VT 05676
(802) 241–2400

Virginia

Virginia Health Care Campaign
Cora Tucker
P.O. Box 356
Halifax, VA 24558
(804) 476–7757

Office on Aging
101 North 14th St., 18th Fl.
Richmond, VA 23219
(804) 225–2271

Washington

Bureau of Aging and Adult Services
Department of Social and Health
  Services, OB-43G
Olympia, WA 98504
(206) 753–2502

Affordable Health Care Campaign
Jessica Schubach
1205 E. Pike Ave., Rm. 2C
Seattle, WA 98122
(206) 329–9764

Evergreen Legal Services
Ada Sneen-Jaffe
101 Yesler Way, #300
Seattle, WA 98104
(206) 464–5933

Washington Fair Share
Dwight Pelz, director
1205 E. Pike, Rm. 2C
Seattle, WA 98122
(206) 329–9764

West Virginia

Commission on Aging
State Capitol
Charleston, WV 25305
(304) 348–3317

West Virginia Citizen Action Group
David Grubb
1324 Virginia St., East
Charleston, WV 25301
(304) 346–5891

West Virginia Legal Services Plan
James P. Martin
1033 Quarrier St., Ste. 700
Charleston, WV 25301
(304) 342–6814

Wisconsin

Bureau on Aging
1 West Wilson St., Room 685
Madison, WI 53702
(608) 272–8606

Legal Action of Wisconsin
Thomas Dixon
31 South Mills Street

Madison, WI 53715
(608) 256–3304

Wisconsin Action Coalition
Jeff Eagan, director
152 West Wisconsin Ave., Suite 633
Milwaukee, WI 53203
(414) 272–2562

Wyoming

Legal Services of SE Wyoming, Inc.
Robert A. Oakley

1620 Capitol Ave., #200
Cheyenne, WY 82001
(307) 634–1566

Wyoming Commission on Aging
Hathaway Building, #139
Cheyenne, WY 82002
(307) 777–7986

Appendix H

Local AIDS-Related Groups

Note: These listings were adapted by the author from the most recent (1988) membership directory of the National AIDS Network (NAN), which is the national "association" of all local AIDS-related groups and agencies; organizations formed or reorganized since early 1988—or organizations which have not affiliated with NAN—have no other mechanism to become "known" for any national listing. Thus, local areas often have a number of AIDS service organizations not listed here. Local agencies which *are* listed in this directory can acquaint the interested reader with additional, unlisted area groups.

Alabama
Birmingham: AIDS Outreach (205) 930–0440; (800) 445–3741
Mobile: AIDS Buddy Program (205) 476–9142; AIDS Coalition (205) 344–5684
Montgomery: AIDS Outreach (205) 284–2273
Tuscaloosa: West Alabama AIDS Network (205) 345–0067

Alaska
Anchorage: Alaska AIDS Project (907) 276–4880; (800) 478–AIDS

Arizona
Phoenix: Arizona AIDS Project (602) 277–1929
Tucson: AIDS Project (602) 322–6226; (602) 326–AIDS

Arkansas
Little Rock: AIDS Foundation (501) 224–4020; (501) 374–5503

California
Bakersfield: AIDS Task Force (805) 328–0729
Berkeley: Gay Men's Health Collective (415) 644–0425
Campbell: Aris Project (408) 370–3272
Concord: Diablo V Community Church (415) 827–2960
Fresno: Central Valley AIDS Team (209) 264–2437
Garden Grove: AIDS Response Program (714) 534–0862
Guerneville: Face to Face (707) 887–1581
Irvine: Buddhist AIDS Project (213) 859–5536

Long Beach: Project Ahead (213) 439–3948
Los Angeles: AIDS Project (213) 962–1600; (213) 876–AIDS
Merced: AIDS Support Team (209) 385–7709
Modesto: Stanislaus Community AIDS Project (209) 572–2437
Oakland: AIDS Project of the East Bay (415) 420–8181
Palm Springs: Desert AIDS Project-CCCC, Inc. (619) 323–2118
Redding: North State AIDS Project (916) 225–5252
Sacramento: AIDS Foundation (916) 448–2437
San Diego: AIDS Assistance Fund (619) 543–0300; AIDS Project (619) 543–0300
San Francisco: AIDS Benefits Counselors (415) 673–3780; AIDS Foundation (415)
    864–4376, (800) FOR–AIDS; Balif AIDS Legal Referral Panel (415) 864–8186;
    Shanti Project (415) 777–2273
San Luis Obispo: AIDS Task Force (805) 549–5540
Santa Barbara: Tri-Counties AIDS Project (805) 681–5120
Santa Cruz: AIDS Project (408) 458–4999
Santa Rosa: Sonoma County AIDS Project (707) 527–2247
West Hollywood: AIDS Project (213) 876–8951; Shanti Foundation (213) 273–7591

Colorado
Denver: Colorado AIDS Project (303) 837–0166

Connecticut
Bantam: N.W. Connecticut AIDS Project (203) 482–1596; (203) 567–4111
Hartford: Gay/Lesbian Health Collective (203) 236–4431
New Britain: AIDS Project (203) 225–7634; (203) 225–6789
New Haven: AIDS Project (203) 624–2437

District of Columbia
Washington: Damien Ministries (202) 387–2926; Lifelink (202) 833–3070;
    Whitman-Walker Clinic (202) 797–3500

Delaware
Wilmington: Delaware Lesbian and Gay Health Advocates AIDS Co.
(302) 652–6776

Florida
Daytona Beach: DARE (904) 257–4028
Ft. Lauderdale: AIDS Center One (305) 561–0316; (800) 325–5371
Key West: AIDS Help Inc. (305) 296–6196
Lakeland: Polk AIDS Support Service (813) 665–7071
Miami: Health Crisis Network (305) 326–8833; (305) 634–4636
Orlando: Central Florida AIDS Unified Resources, Inc. (305) 849–1452
Sarasota: AIDS Support (813) 951–1551
Tampa: AIDS Network (813) 221–6420; (813) 221–6420

Georgia
Athens: AIDS Support Group (404) 546–0737
Atlanta: AID Atlanta (404) 872–0600; (800) 551–2728
Macon: Central City AIDS Network (912) 742–2437
Savannah: First City Network, Inc. (912) 236–CITY

Hawaii
Honolulu: Life Foundation (808) 924–2437
Kailua: Hawaii Council of Churches (808) 263–9788
Volcano: AIDS Helpline (808) 967–7202

Idaho
Boise: Idaho AIDS Foundation (208) 345–2277

Illinois
Belleville: Helping Hands of Southern Illinois (618) 234–9365
Champaign: Champaign AIDS (217) 351–2437
Chicago: AIDS Education Project (312) 908–9191; AIDS Foundation
(312) 525–9466; Howard Brown Memorial Clinic (312) 871–5777

Indiana
Evansville: AIDS Resource Group (812) 423–7791
Fort Wayne: AIDS Task Force (219) 484–2711
Indianapolis: AIDS Task Force (317) 634–1441; (317) 257–HOPE

Iowa
Des Moines: Central Iowa AIDS Project (800) 445–AIDS
Iowa City: Iowa Center For AIDS/ARC Education (319) 351–0140
Waterloo: AIDS Coalition of Northeast Iowa (319) 234–6831

Kansas
Topeka: Kansas AIDS Network (800) 247–4101; (800) 247–7499; AIDS Project
   (913) 232–3100
Wichita: AIDS Project (316) 267–1852

Kentucky
Lexington: AIDS Crisis Taskforce (606) 281–5151
Louisville: Community Health Trust (502) 636–3341; (502) 637–4342

Louisiana
Baton Rouge: MCC-AIDS Project (504) 387–4424
New Orleans: NO/AIDS Task Force (504) 891–3732; (800) 992–4379

Maine
Portland: AIDS Project (207) 774–6877; (800) 851–AIDS

Maryland

Baltimore: H.E.R.O. (301) 685–1180; (800) 638–6252
Rockville: Montgomery County HERO (301) 762–3385
Silver Spring: African Center AIDS Project (301) 622–0129

Massachusetts

Boston: AIDS Action (617) 437–6200; (800) 235–2331
Brighton: Project Win (617) 783–7300
Cambridge: AIDS Family Support Group (617) 491–0600

Michigan

Detroit: AIDS Phone Network (313) 567–1640
Ferndale: PWA Food Bank (313) 864–3740
Grand Rapids: AIDS Task Force (616) 956–9009
Hamtramck: Friends, People with AIDS Alliance (313) 365–2450

Minnesota

Minneapolis: Minnesota AIDS Project (612) 870–7773; (800) 248–AIDS

Mississippi

Jackson: Mississippi Gay Alliance (601) 353–7611

Missouri

Columbia: MID Missouri AIDS Project (314) 875–2437
Kansas City: Good Samaritan Project (816) 561–8784
St. Louis: Effort For AIDS (314) 531–2847; (314) 531–7400
Springfield: AIDS Project/Springfield (417) 864–8373

Montana

Billings: AIDS Support Network (406) 252–1212

Nebraska

Omaha: Nebraska AIDS Project (402) 342–4233; Project Concern/AIDS Coalition
  (402) 455–3701

Nevada

Las Vegas: Aid for AIDS of Nevada (702) 369–6162
Reno: Nevada AIDS Foundation (702) 329–2437

New Hampshire

Concord: New Hampshire Buddy System (603) 595–0218
Manchester: New Hampshire AIDS Foundation (603) 753–9533

New Jersey

Neptune: AIDS Information Group (201) 758–0077
New Brunswick: AIDS Foundation (201) 992–5666; (201) 246–0925
Newark: New Jersey Lesbian & Gay AIDS Awareness (201) 596–0767
Randolph: Interfaith AIDS (201) 895–4874
Vineland: Casa Prac, Inc. (609) 692–2331

New Mexico
Albuquerque: New Mexico AIDS Services (505) 266–0911

New York
Albany: AIDS Council (518) 434–4686; (518) 445–AIDS
Bridgehampton: East End Gay Organization (516) 537–2480; (516) 385–AIDS
Bronx: Pediatric AIDS Hotline (212) 430–4227; (212) 430–3333
Brooklyn: AIDS Task Force C.S.P. (718) 596–4781
Buffalo: Western New York AIDS Program (716) 847–2441; (716) 847–AIDS
Johnson City: Southern Tier AIDS Program, Inc. (607) 723–6520
New York: Gay Men's Health Crisis (212) 807–6664; (212) 807–6655
Richmond Hill: AIDS Center (718) 575–8855
Rochester: AIDS Rochester, Inc. (716) 232–3580; (716) 232–4430
Syracuse: AIDS Task Force (315) 475–2430; (315) 875–AIDS
White Plains: Mid-Hudson Valley AIDS Task Force (914) 993–0606

North Carolina
Asheville: Western North Carolina AIDS Project (704) 252–7489
Charlotte: Metrolina AIDS Project (704) 333–2437
Durham: Lesbian & Gay Health Project (919) 683–2182
Greensboro: Triad Health Project (919) 275–1654
Greenville: Eastern Regional AIDS Support (919) 355–4568
Raleigh: AIDS Control Program (919) 733–7301
Wilmington: Grow AIDS Resource Project (919) 675–9222
Winston-Salem: AIDS Task Force (919) 723–5031

Ohio
Akron: AIDS Task Force (216) 375–2960
Canton: AIDS Task Force (216) 489–3231
Cincinnati: Ambrose Clement Health Clinic (513) 352–3139
Cleveland: Health Issues Task Force (216) 621–0766
Columbus: AIDS Task Force (614) 224–0411
Portsmouth: Southern Ohio AIDS Task Force (614) 353–3339
Toledo: Area AIDS Task Force, Inc. (419) 243–9351
Youngstown: AIDS Task Force (216) 742–8700

Oklahoma
Oklahoma City: Oasis Community Center (405) 525–AIDS

Oregon
Eugene: Willamette AIDS Council (503) 345–7089
Portland: Cascade AIDS Project (503) 223–5907; (800) 777–AIDS; Oregon AIDS
    Task Force (503) 226–6678

Pennsylvania
Allentown: AIDS Service Center (215) 435–4616
Altoona: AIDS Intervention Project (814) 946–5411; (800) 445–6262

Chester: American Red Cross (215) 874–1484
Harrisburg: South Central AIDS Assistance Network (717) 236–4772
Lancaster: AIDS Project (717) 394–3380; (717) 394–9900
Philadelphia: Action AIDS (215) 732–2155; AIDS Task Force (215) 545–8686;
   (215) 732–AIDS
Pittsburgh: AIDS Task Force (412) 363–6500; (412) 363–2437
Reading: Berks AIDS Health Crisis (215) 375–2242
Scranton: North East AIDS Council (717) 342–4562

Rhode Island
Providence: Project AIDS (401) 277–6545; (401) 277–6502

South Carolina
Columbia: Carolina AIDS Research and Education (803) 777–2273

South Dakota
Sioux Falls: Sioux Empire Gay & Lesbian Coalition (605) 332–4599

Tennessee
Chattanooga: Chattanooga Cares (615) 265–2273
Knoxville: AIDS Response (615) 523–2437; (615) 523–AIDS
Memphis: Aids to End AIDS Committee (901) 454–1411
Nashville: Nashville Cares (615) 385–1510; (615) 385–AIDS

Texas
Austin: AIDS Service (512) 458–AIDS
Dallas: AIDS Resource Center (214) 521–5124; (214) 559–AIDS
El Paso: Southwest AIDS Committee (915) 533–6809; (915) 541–4266
Houston: AIDS Foundation (713) 623–6796
San Antonio: AIDS Foundation (512) 733–1853

Vermont
Burlington: Vermont Cares (802) 863–2437

Virginia
Charlottesville: AIDS Support Group (804) 979–7714
Norfolk: Tidewater AIDS Crisis Taskforce (804) 423–5859
Richmond: AIDS Information (804) 355–4428; (804) 358–6343

Washington
Seattle: Northwest AIDS Foundation (206) 329–6923; AIDS Action Committee
   (206) 323–1229

Wisconsin
Milwaukee: AIDS Project (414) 273–2437; (800) 334–2437

Appendix I

Foreclosure Prevention Programs Available to Homeowners with Governmentally Insured Mortgages
by Robert F. Gillett

Procedures and Defenses: Government-Insured Mortgages

(Note: Statutory, regulatory, and procedural provisions related in this paper were those in effect as of 1985, with major substantive changes through mid-1989 noted in minor textual revisions. In late 1989, HUD Secretary Kemp announced plans to "tighten" FHA mortgage insurance regulations; such changes might affect the provisions discussed below. PWAs and their advocates who face mortgage delinquency should seek the advice of an attorney, banker, or realtor with technical expertise in mortgage/real estate matters before exploring remedies discussed below.)

I. Foreclosures on FHA- and HUD-Insured Mortgages.
Clients with FHA- and HUD-insured mortgages have significant rights not available to persons with uninsured loans.
   (A) Mortgage servicing efforts (by private mortgagee) 24 CFR 203.600, et seq., HUD Handbook, 4330.1.
      1. *Foreclosure.*
      Mortgagee cannot commence foreclosure for a monetary default unless at least three (3) full monthly installments are due. 24 CFR 203.650(a)(2).
      2. *Reinstatement.* 24 CFR 203.608.
         (a) Mortgagee shall permit reinstatement even after the institution of foreclosure proceedings if the mortgagor tenders the full amount due including foreclosure costs and reasonable attorney's fees.
         (b) But, if the mortgagee has, within the past two (2) years, accepted a reinstatement after initiation of foreclosure proceedings, the mortgagee need not stop the foreclosure.

Source: Excerpted here by permission of Robert F. Gillett.

3. *Forbearance.* 24 CFR 203.614.

   (a) Lending institutions may grant forbearance without HUD approval if the default was caused by circumstances beyond the mortgagor's control.

     (1) Agreement between mortgagor and lending institution must provide for:

       (i) Suspension or reduction of payments for a period not exceeding eighteen (18) months;

       (ii) Resumption of regular mortgage payments after the expiration of the period of reduced or suspended payments; and

       (iii) Repayment of the total unpaid amount accruing prior to and during the period of reduced or suspended payments on or before a date extending beyond the original maturity date for a period no longer than the period of forbearance.

   (b) HUD may approve forbearance relief itself if it finds that the default was caused by circumstances beyond the mortgagor's control. In this case, lending institution and mortgagor must sign an agreement providing for:

     (1) The increase, reduction or suspension of payments for a specified forbearance period;

     (2) The resumption of regular monthly payments after expiration of the forbearance period; and

     (3) The payment of the total unpaid amount accruing prior to and during the forbearance period on or before the maturity date of the mortgage.

4. *Recasting. See* 24 CFR 203.616.

   (a) The Secretary may also approve a modification of mortgage by recasting the delinquency over the remaining term of the mortgage or over such longer period of time as the Secretary may approve.

   (b) Where the lender determines that the buyer does not own other property subject to a mortgage insured by the Secretary, the lender may recast the mortgage without obtaining HUD's approval. In such instances the recasting shall not extend more than ten (10) years beyond the original maturity date. HUD shall be given notice of the modification within thirty (30) days after the execution of the modification agreement.

5. *Procedural Protections.*

   (a) Mortgagee must give notice to a mortgagor in default on a form supplied by HUD. 24 CFR 203.602. This notice must be given no later than the end of the second month of delinquency. The lender is not required to send a second delinquency notice to the same mortgagor more than once each six (6) months. *See* 24 CFR 203.602.

(b) Mortgagee must have a face-to-face interview with the mortgagor, or make a reasonable effort to arrange such a meeting, before three (3) full monthly installments due on the mortgage are unpaid. 24 CFR 203.604(b). What is a reasonable effort? It is at a minimum one letter sent to the mortgagor by certified mail and at least one trip to see the mortgagor at the mortgaged property. 24 CFR 203.604(d). *But see* 24 CFR 203.604(c).

(B) The HUD Mortgage Assignment Program.
Individuals who have mortgages insured under Sections 203, 221, or 235 of the National Housing Act and who default on their mortgage payments may, in certain circumstances, qualify for assignment of the mortgage to HUD and postponement of payments for up to thirty-six (36) months. 24 CFR 203.600, et seq.; *see* 24 CFR 221.251 and 24 CFR 235.1. *See* Handbook 4330.2.

1. HUD will accept assignment of mortgage to avoid foreclosure if the following conditions are met:
   (a) Mortgagee has given notice of foreclosure to mortgagor;
   (b) At least three (3) monthly installments are due;
   (c) The property is the mortgagor's principal place of residence;
   (d) The default has been caused by circumstances beyond the mortgagor's control which render the mortgagor unable to correct the delinquency within a reasonable time or make full mortgage payments;
   (e) There is a reasonable prospect that the mortgagor will be able to resume full mortgage payments after a temporary period of reduced or suspended payments not exceeding thirty-six (36) months and will be able to pay the mortgage in full by its maturity date extended, if necessary, by up to ten (10) years; *see* 24 CFR 203.650.

2. Assignment Procedures
   (a) The lending institution must notify the mortgagor that he is in default, that the mortgagee intends to foreclose unless the mortgagor cures the default, and that the mortgagee is considering whether to request HUD to accept assignment. 24 CFR 203.651.
   (b) Second, the lending institution determines whether the criteria necessary for assignment are present. 24 CFR 203.652.
   (c) Third, if the lending institution determines that all of the assignment criteria are not met, it must advise the mortgagor that he/she may request HUD to accept assignment. 24 CFR 203.652(b).
   (d) Fourth, the mortgagor must contact HUD within fifteen (15) days after the lending institution's notice. 24 CFR 203.652(b).
   (e) Fifth, HUD decides whether or not to accept assignment. If HUD decides against acceptance of the assignment, it must notify the mortgagor of the reasons. 24 CFR 203.654(b) and (c).

      (f) If HUD denies a request for assignment:

          (1) The mortgagor has fifteen (15) days in which to present additional information or

          (2) The mortgagor may, within twenty (20) days of HUD's initial determination, present his/her case at a personal conference with a HUD representative. 24 CFR 203.654 (c).

          (3) HUD shall promptly notify the mortgagor of its decision and, if it decides against assignment, it must give the reasons for its decision. 24 CFR 203.658.

      (g) The lending institution should not initiate foreclosure before the mortgagor has had an opportunity to request of HUD that it accept assignment. 24 CFR 203.658.

(C) HUD-Occupied Conveyance Program. 24 CFR 203.670, et seq. HUD Handbook 4310.5. (Note: Regulations on this program have been rewritten since 1985, and the approval rate for occupied conveyances has consequently been significantly reduced.)

  1. After foreclosure HUD may permit a foreclosed mortgagor (or a tenant of a foreclosed mortgagor) to remain in the premises and rent from HUD.

  2. *Eligibility.* An occupant will be considered for the occupied conveyance program if:

      (a) It is in HUD's interest to accept occupied conveyance; that is, that because of a higher neighborhood vacancy rate or a vandalism problem in the area, HUD's financial interest in the property will be protected by continued occupancy. 24 CFR 203.671.

      (b) An occupant may be permitted to remain in the premises when the "Secretary's interest" criteria is not met, where the occupant or a member of her family suffers from a temporary illness or injury which would be aggravated by the moving process. *See* 24 CFR 203.670 (a)(2).

      (c) The property is habitable. *See* CFR 203.675. (This is a lower standard of habitability than a code compliance standard.)

      (d) The applicant has resided in the property for sixty (60) days. 24 CFR 203.674(a).

      (e) The occupant has the financial ability to make monthly rental payments, and agrees to execute a lease and pay one month's rent in advance. 24 CFR 203.674(c), (d) and (e).

  3. *Occupied Conveyance Process.*

      (a) Between sixty to ninety (60-90) days prior to the date that the mortgagee expects to acquire title, the mortgagee must notify HUD and include, in that notice, the name of the occupant. 24 CFR 203.675.

      (b) HUD notifies the occupant of the availability of the program. 24 CFR 203.676.

(c) The occupant must apply in writing to HUD for consideration for the program within twenty (20) days. 24 CFR 203.676(c).

(d) HUD must provide written reasons for any denial. 24 CFR 203.677.

(e) The occupant may request reconsideration of HUD's denial at a personal conference (within ten (10) days) or by submission of additional information in writing (within twenty (20) days). 26 CFR 203.677(b).

(f) HUD must provide written reasons for any final denial. 24 CFR 203.678.

4. *Resale of HUD-Owned Property.*

(a) The occupied conveyance program is viewed by HUD as a "sale enhancement" program, and the occupant's right to continued possession is subject to HUD's right to sale. 24 CFR 203.680.

(b) The occupant is normally given the right of first refusal on the resale of the property. The purchase price to a foreclosed mortgagor is normally one hundred five percent (105%) of the foreclosure sale price. The occupant must deposit ten percent (10%) of the price in cash with HUD within twenty (20) days of receipt of the notice of sale. FHA-insured financing is normally not available on repurchase. HUD Handbook 4310.5, Chapter 10.

. . . .

III. Foreclosures on VA-Insured Mortgages

Clients with mortgages insured by the VA have rights unavailable to one whose mortgage is a private conventional mortgage but those rights are far more limited than the FHA or FMHA programs. 38 USC 1801, et seq.; 38 CFR 36.4301, et seq.; VA pamphlet 26–7.

(A) VA-insured mortgages may be serviced by the VA or by private mortgagees. A private mortgagee cannot commence foreclosure for a monetary default unless at least three (3) full monthly payments are due. 38 CFR 36.4316(a).

(B) Reinstatement. 38 CFR 36.4308(g).

1. Mortgagee shall permit reinstatement at any time prior to a judicial or statutory sale if the full amount of the delinquency is tendered including installment payments, late charges and reasonable expenses incurred and paid by the holder if the foreclosure has begun.

(C) Extensions and Reamortizations. 38 CFR 36.4314.

1. In the event of default, or to avoid imminent default, the term of the mortgage may be extended by written agreement between the holder and the debtor.

2. Unless there is prior approval of the VA, the terms of the mortgage extension agreement must provide that eighty percent (80%) of the mortgage is amortized within the original time frames.

(D) Partial payments. 38 CFR 36.4315.

1. Partial payments must be accepted up until foreclosure is commenced. The exceptions are contained at 38 CFR 36.4315 (b)(2).

(E) Procedure to be followed in case of default.
1. Mortgagee must give notice to the administrator of the VA of a default and of its intention to foreclose. 38 CFR 36.4317.
2. The mortgagee cannot begin foreclosure proceedings until thirty (30) days after it delivers notice of intention to foreclose.

(F) Refunding of Loans in Default.
1. Authority exists to refund the unpaid balance of the loan or to take an assignment of the loan and the mortgage. 38 USC 1816(a). The regulations provide that within thirty (30) days after receiving notice of intention to default, the administrator may take an assignment. 38 CFR 36.4318. However, because VA regulations do not set forth explicit procedures for addressing and handling this authority, neither mortgagors nor mortgagees are informed of the criteria for relief, basis for or notice of the decision on assignment, offered specific method to apply for relief, given a forum to present facts and evidence in support of relief or given an expressed appeal avenue to contest a denial. Nevertheless, PWAs and their advocates should definitely contact VA officials, in writing, citing the statute and regulation, to invoke refund/assignment rights and aggressively "appeal" an adverse response (or nonresponse) to the highest level in the Department (and, then, the courts).

(G) Supplemental Loans. 38 CFR 36.4355.
1. The VA has the authority to issue supplemental loans for renovation or improvement of insured homes. Existing loans may be consolidated with the new loans. 38 CFR 36.4355.

(H) Rental. Handbook 26–7, Section H, paragraph 11.
1. While the general preference is for property to be vacant before the VA accepts title, the VA may accept conveyance of the property with a rental agreement with the current occupant.

Appendix J

State Vital Statistics Agencies

These state offices handle requests for birth and death certificates. To secure copies of marriage certificates, write to the local official or office which issued the license; for adoption, divorce, separation, custody, or child support decrees, write to the clerk of the court which issued the order.

Most of the states require the following information:
- Full name, sex, and race of the person
- Parents' names, including maiden name of mother
- The month, day, and year of birth or death and the place where it occurred
- Your relationship to the individual and why you need the document.

Alabama
Department of Public Health
Bureau of Vital Statistics
State Office Building
Montgomery, AL 36130
(205) 261–5033
  Fee: $5.00

Alaska
Department of Health & Social Services
Bureau of Vital Statistics
Pouch H–02G
Juneau, AK 99811
(907) 465–3391
  Fee: $5.00

Arizona
Arizona Department of Health Services
Vital Records Section
P.O. Box 3887
Phoenix, AZ 85030
(602) 255–1080
  Fee: $5.00

Arkansas
Arkansas Department of Health
Division of Vital Records
4815 West Markham Street
Little Rock, AR 72201
(501) 661–2336
  Fee: $5.00

California
Department of Health Services
Office of the State Registrar of Vital Statistics
410 N Street
Sacramento, CA 95814
(901) 445–2684
  Fee: $11.00

Colorado
Colorado Department of Health
Vital Records Section
4210 East 11th Avenue
Denver, CO 80220
(303) 320–8474
  Fee: $6.00

Connecticut
Department of Health Services
Vital Records Section
150 Washington Street
Hartford, CT 06106
(203) 566–1124
    Fee: $3.00

Delaware
Office of Vital Statistics
Robbins Building
P.O. Box 637
Dover, DE 19903
(302) 736–4721
    Fee: $5.00

District of Columbia
Vital Records Branch
425 I Street, N.W., Room 3009
Washington, DC 20001
(202) 727–5316
    Fee: $5.00

Florida
Department of Health and Rehabilitative
    Services
Office of Vital Statistics
P.O. Box 210
Jacksonville, FL 32231
(904) 359–6900
    Fee: $6.50

Georgia
Georgia Department of Human
    Resources
Vital Records Unit
Room 217–H
47 Trinity Avenue, S.W.
Atlanta, GA 30334
(404) 656–4900
    Fee: $3.00

Hawaii
Research and Statistics Office
State Department of Health
P.O. Box 3378

Honolulu, HI 96801
(808) 548–5819
    Fee: $2.00

Idaho
Department of Health & Welfare
Bureau of Vital Statistics, Standards &
    Local Health Services
450 West State Street
Boise, ID 83720
(208) 334–5988
    Fee: $6.00

Illinois
Illinois Department of Health
Division of Vital Records
605 West Jefferson Street
Springfield, IL 62702
(217) 782–6553
    Fee: $15.00

Indiana
Indiana State Board of Health
Division of Vital Records
1330 West Michigan Street
P.O. Box 1964
Indianapolis, IN 46206
(317) 633–0274
    Fee: $6.00

Iowa
Iowa Department of Public Health
Vital Records Section
Lucas State Office Building
Des Moines, IA 50319
(515) 281–5871
    Fee: $6.00

Kansas
Department of Health & Environment
Office of Vital Statistics
900 Jackson Street
Topeka, KS 66612
(913) 296–1400
    Fee: $6.00

Kentucky
Department of Health Services
Office of Vital Statistics
275 East Main Street
Frankfort, KY 40621
(502) 564–4212
  Fee: $5.00

Louisiana
Division of Vital Records
Office of Health Services and
  Environmental Quality
P.O. Box 60630
New Orleans, LA 70160
(504) 568–5175
  Fee: $8.00

Maine
Office of Vital Statistics
State House, Station 11
221 State Street
Augusta, ME 04333
(207) 289–3181
  Fee: $5.00

Maryland
Department of Health & Mental Hygiene
Division of Vital Records
P.O. Box 13146
201 West Preston Street
Baltimore, MD 21203
(301) 225–5988
  Fee: $3.00

Massachusetts
Department of Public Health
Registry of Vital Records & Statistics
150 Tremont Street, Room B–3
Boston, MA 02111
(617) 727–0110
  Fee: $3.00

Michigan
Department of Public Health
Office of the State Registrar & Center
  for Health Statistics

3500 North Logan Street
Lansing, MI 48090
(517) 335–8655
  Fee: $10.00

Minnesota
Minnesota Department of Health
Vital Records Section
717 Delaware Street, S.E.
P.O. Box 9441
Minneapolis, MN 55440
(612) 623–5121
  Fee: $11.00

Mississippi
Mississippi State Board of Health
Vital Records
P.O. Box 1700
Jackson, MS 39215
(601) 354–6606
  Fee: $10.00

Missouri
Department of Health
Bureau of Vital Records
P.O. Box 570
Jefferson City, MO 65102
(314) 751–6387
  Fee: $4.00

Montana
Department of Health and
  Environmental Sciences
Bureau of Records & Statistics
Cogswell Building
Helena, MT 59620
(406) 444–2614
  Fee: $5.00

Nebraska
Department of Health
Bureau of Vital Statistics
301 Centennial Mall South
P.O. Box 95007
Lincoln, NE 68509
(402) 471–2871
  Fee: $6.00

Nevada
Department of Human Resources
Division of Health
Capitol Complex
505 East King Street
Carson City, NV 89710
(702) 885–4480
Fee: $6.00

New Hampshire
Bureau of Vital Records
Health & Human Services Building
6 Hazen Drive
Concord, NH 03301
(603) 271–4654
Fee: $3.00

New Jersey
Department of Health
Bureau of Vital Statistics
CN 360
Trenton, NJ 08625
(609) 292–4087
Fee: $4.00

New Mexico
Vital Statistics Bureau
New Mexico Health Services Division
P.O. Box 968
Santa Fe, NM 87504
(505) 827–2338
Fee: $10.00

New York *(except New York City)*
State Department of Health
Bureau of Vital Records
Empire State Plaza
Tower Building
Albany, NY 12237
(518) 474–3075
Fee: $5.00

New York City
New York City Department of Health
Bureau of Vital Records
125 Worth Street

New York, NY 10013
(212) 619–4530
Fee: $5.00

North Carolina
Department of Human Resources
Division of Health Service
Vital Records Branch
P.O. Box 2091
Raleigh, NC 27602
(919) 733–3526
Fee: $5.00

North Dakota
State Department of Health
Division of Vital Records
State Capitol, Judicial Wing
Bismarck, ND 58505
(701) 224–2360
Fee: $7.00

Ohio
Ohio Department of Health
Division of Vital Statistics
65 South Front Street, Room G–20
Columbus, OH 43266
(614) 466–2531
Fee: $7.00

Oklahoma
Vital Records Section
State Department of Health
Northeast 10th Street & Stonewall
P.O. Box 53551
Oklahoma City, OK 73152
(405) 271–4040
Fee: $5.00

Oregon
Department of Human Resources
Health Division, Vital Records Section
P.O. Box 116
Portland, OR 97207
(503) 229–5710
Fee: $8.00

Pennsylvania
Department of Health
Division of Vital Records
101 South Mercer Street
P.O. Box 1528
New Castle, PA 16103
(412) 656–3100
  Fee: $4.00

Rhode Island
Department of Health
Division of Vital Statistics
Room 101, Cannon Building
75 Davis Street
Providence, RI 02908
(401) 277–2811
  Fee: $5.00

South Carolina
Dept. of Health & Environmental
  Control
Office of Vital Records & Public Health
  Statistics
2600 Bull Street
Columbia, SC 29201
(803) 734–4830
  Fee: $5.00

South Dakota
Department of Health
Center for Health Statistics
Joe Foss Building
523 East Capitol
Pierre, SD 57501
(605) 773–3355
  Fee: $5.00

Tennessee
Tennessee Vital Records
Department of Health and Environment
Cordell Hull Building
Nashville, TN 37219
(615) 741–1763
(800) 423–1901 (TN only)
  Fee: $6.00

Texas
Texas Department of Health
Bureau of Vital Statistics
1100 West 49th Street
Austin, TX 78756
(512) 458–7380
  Fee: $5.00

Utah
Utah Department of Health
Bureau of Vital Records
288 North 1460 West
P.O. Box 16700
Salt Lake City, UT 84116
(801) 538–6105
  Fee: $10.00

Vermont
Vermont Department of Health
Vital Records Section
P.O. Box 70
60 Main Street
Burlington, VT 05402
(802) 863–7275
  Fee: $5.00

Virginia
Department of Health
Division of Vital Records
James Madison Building
P.O. Box 1000
Richmond, VA 23208
(804) 786–6228
  Fee: $5.00

Virgin Islands
Bureau of Vital Statistics
Department of Health
P.O. Box 520 C'sted.
St. Croix, VI 00820
(809) 773–4050
  Fee: $5.00

Washington
Department of Social & Health Services
Vital Records

P.O. Box 9709, ET–11
Olympia, WA 98504
(206) 753–5396
(800) 331–0680 (in state)
(800) 551–0562 (out of state)
  Fee: $6.00

West Virginia
Department of Health
Division of Vital Statistics
State Office Building No. 3
Charleston, WV 25305
(304) 348–2931
  Fee: $5.00

Wisconsin
Bureau of Health Statistics
Division of Health
1 West Wilson Street
P.O. Box 309
Madison, WI 53701
(608) 266–1371
  Fee: $7.00

Wyoming
Vital Records Services
Division of Health & Medical Services
Hathaway Building
Cheyenne, WY 82002
(307) 777–7591
  Fee: $5.00

Appendix K

State Insurance Agencies

Alabama
Commissioner of Insurance
135 South Union Street, #181
Montgomery, AL 36130
(205) 269–3550

Alaska
Director of Insurance
P.O. Box "D"
Juneau, AK 99811
(907) 465–2515

Arizona
Director of Insurance
801 East Jefferson, 2nd Floor
Phoenix, AZ 85034
(602) 255–4367

Arkansas
Insurance Commissioner
400 University Tower Building
12th & University Streets
Little Rock, AR 72204
(501) 371–1325

California
Commissioner of Insurance
100 Van Ness Avenue
San Francisco, CA 94102
(415) 557–3245 (San Francisco)
(213) 736–2551 (Los Angeles)
(800) 233–9045 (rest of state)

Colorado
Commissioner of Insurance
303 West Colfax Ave., 5th Floor
Denver, CO 80204
(303) 866–3201

Connecticut
Insurance Commissioner
165 Capitol Avenue
State Office Building, Room 425
Hartford, CT 06106
(203) 736–4251

Delaware
Insurance Commissioner
841 Silver Lake Boulevard
Dover, DE 19901
(302) 736–4251

District of Columbia
Superintendent of Insurance
614 H Street, N.W., Suite 516
Washington, DC 20001
(202) 727–7419

Florida
Insurance Commissioner
State Capitol Plaza, Level 11
Tallahassee, FL 32399
(904) 488–3440

Georgia
Insurance Commissioner
2 Martin Luther King, Jr. Drive

704 West Tower
Atlanta, GA 30334
(404) 656–2056

Hawaii
Insurance Commissioner
P.O. Box 3614
Honolulu, HI 96811
(808) 548–5450

Idaho
Director of Insurance
700 West State Street
Boise, ID 83720
(208) 334–2250

Illinois
Director of Insurance
320 West Washington St., 4th Floor
Springfield, IL 62767
(217) 782–4515

Indiana
Commissioner of Insurance
311 West Washington St., Suite 300
Indianapolis, IN 46204
(317) 232–2386

Iowa
Commissioner of Insurance
Lucas State Office Bldg., 6th Floor
Des Moines, IA 50319
(515) 281–5705

Kansas
Commissioner of Insurance
420 S.W. 9th Street
Topeka, KS 66612
(913) 296–7801

Kentucky
Insurance Commissioner
229 West Main St., P.O. Box 517
Frankfort, KY 40602
(502) 564–3630

Louisiana
Commissioner of Insurance
P.O. Box 44214
Baton Rouge, LA 70804
(504) 342–5328

Maine
Superintendent of Insurance
State Office Building
State House, Station 34
Augusta, ME 04333
(207) 289–3101

Maryland
Insurance Commissioner
501 St. Paul Place
Stanbalt Building, 7th Floor South
Baltimore, MD 21202
(301) 333–2520

Massachusetts
Commissioner of Insurance
100 Cambridge Street
Boston, MA 02202
(617) 727–3333

Michigan
Insurance Commissioner
P.O. Box 30220
Lansing, MI 48909
(517) 373–9273

Minnesota
Commissioner of Commerce
500 Metro Square Bldg., 5th Floor
St. Paul, MN 55101
(612) 296–6907

Mississippi
Commissioner of Insurance
1804 Walter Sillers Bldg.
P.O. Box 79
Jackson, MS 39205
(601) 359–3569

Missouri
Director of Insurance
301 West High St., 6 North
P.O. Box 690
Jefferson City, MO 65102
(314) 751–2451

Montana
Commissioner of Insurance
126 North Sanders Mitchell Bldg.
Room 270, P.O. Box 4009
Helena, MT 59601
(406) 444–2040

Nebraska
Director of Insurance
301 Centennial Mall, South
P.O. Box 94699
Lincoln, NE 68509
(402) 471–2201

Nevada
Commissioner of Insurance
Nye Bldg., 201 South Fall Street
Carson City, NV 89701
(702) 885–4270

New Hampshire
Insurance Commissioner
169 Manchester Street
P.O. Box 2005
Concord, NH 03301
(603) 271–2261

New Jersey
Commissioner of Insurance
201 East State Street
Trenton, NJ 08625
(609) 292–5363

New Mexico
Superintendent of Insurance
PERA Building, P.O. Drawer 12
Santa Fe, NM 87504
(505) 827–4500

New York
Superintendent of Insurance
160 West Broadway
New York, NY 10013
(212) 602–0429
(800) 342–3736

North Carolina
Commissioner of Insurance
P.O. Box 26387
Raleigh, NC 27611
(919) 733–7343
(800) 662–7777

North Dakota
Commissioner of Insurance
Capitol Building, 5th Floor
Bismarck, ND 58505
(701) 224–2440

Ohio
Director of Insurance
2100 Stella Court
Columbus, OH 43266
(614) 481–5735

Oklahoma
Insurance Commissioner
P.O. Box 53408
Oklahoma City, OK 73152
(405) 521–2828

Oregon
Insurance Commissioner
Labor & Insurance Building
Salem, OR 97310
(503) 378–4271

Pennsylvania
Insurance Commissioner
Strawberry Square, 13th Floor
Harrisburg, PA 17120
(717) 787–5173

Puerto Rico
Commissioner of Insurance
Martinez Juncos Station
Box 8330
Santurce, PR 00910
(809) 722–8686

Rhode Island
Insurance Commissioner
100 North Main Street
Providence, RI 02903
(401) 277–2246

South Carolina
Insurance Commissioner
1612 Marion Street
P.O. Box 100105
Columbia, SC 29202
(803) 737–6117

South Dakota
Insurance Commissioner
Insurance Bldg., 910 East Sioux
Pierre, SD 57501
(605) 773–3563

Tennessee
Commissioner of Insurance
1808 West End Avenue, 14th Floor
Nashville, TN 37219
(615) 741–2241

Texas
Commissioner of Insurance
1110 San Jacinto Building
Austin, TX 78701
(512) 475–3726
(800) 252–3439

Utah
Commissioner of Insurance
P.O. Box 45803
Salt Lake City, UT 84145
(801) 530–6400

Vermont
Commissioner of Insurance
State Office Building
Montpelier, VT 05602
(802) 828–3301

Virginia
Commissioner of Insurance
700 Jefferson Building
P.O. Box 1157
Richmond, VA 23209
(804) 786–3741

Virgin Islands
Commissioner of Insurance
Kongens Garde 18
St. Thomas, VI 00801
(809) 774–2991

Washington
Insurance Commissioner
Insurance Building AQ21
Olympia, WA 98504
(206) 753–7301

West Virginia
Insurance Commissioner
2100 West Street, East
Charleston, WV 25305
(304) 348–3394

Wisconsin
Commissioner of Insurance
P.O. Box 7873
Madison, WI 53707
(608) 266–0102

Wyoming
Insurance Commissioner
Herschler Building
122 West 25th Street
Cheyenne, WY 82002
(307) 777–7401

Appendix L

State Peer Review Organizations (PROs)

Alabama

Alabama Quality Assurance Foundation
236 Goodwin Crest Drive
Suite 300, Twin Towers East
Birmingham, AL 35209
(205) 942–0785

Alaska

Professional Review Organization for
  Washington
2150 North 107th St., Suite 200
Seattle, WA 98133
(206) 364–9700

Arizona

Health Services Advisory Group, Inc.
P.O. Box 16731
Phoenix, AZ 85014
(602) 264–6382

Arkansas

Arkansas Foundation for Medical Care,
  Inc.
809 Garrison Avenue
P.O. Box 1508
Fort Smith, AR 72902
(501) 785–2471

California

California Medical Review, Inc.
1388 Sutter Street, Suite 1100
San Francisco, CA 94109
(415) 923–2000

Colorado

Colorado Foundation for Medical Care
Suite 400, Building 2
6825 East Tennessee Avenue
Denver, CO 80224
(303) 321–8642

Connecticut

Connecticut Peer Review Organization,
  Inc.
384 Pratt Street
Meriden, CT 06450
(203) 237–2773

Delaware

West Virginia Medical Institute, Inc.
3412 Chesterfield Avenue, S.E.
Charleston, WV 25304
(304) 925–0461

District of Columbia

Delmarva Foundation for Medical Care,
  Inc.
341–B North Aurora Street
Easton, MD 21601
(301) 822–0697

Florida

Professional Foundation for Health Care,
  Inc.
2907 Bay to Bay Blvd., Suite 100
Tampa, FL 33629
(813) 831–6273

Georgia
Georgia Medical Care Foundation
4 Executive Park Dr., N.E., Suite 1300
Atlanta, GA 30329
(404) 982–6500

Hawaii
Hawaii Medical Services Association
818 Keeaumoku Street
P.O. Box 860
Honolulu, HI 96808
(808) 944–2110

Idaho
Professional Review Organization for
 Washington
2150 North 107th St., Suite 200
Seattle, WA 98133
(206) 364–9700

Illinois
Crescent Counties Foundation for
 Medical Care
350 Shuman Blvd., Suite 240
Naperville, IL 60540
(312) 876–0652

Indiana
Peerview, Inc.
501 Congressional Blvd., Suite 200
Carmel, IN 40632
(317) 573–6888

Iowa
Iowa Foundation for Medical Care
3737 Woodland Ave., Suite 500
West Des Moines, IA 50265
(515) 223–2900

Kansas
Kansas Foundation for Medical Care,
 Inc.
2947 S.W. Wanamaker Drive
Topeka, KS 66614
(913) 273–2552

Kentucky
Peerview, Inc.
10300 Linn Station Rd., Suite 100
Louisville, KY 40223
(502) 429–0995

Louisiana
Louisiana Health Care Review
9357 Interline Ave., Suite 200
Baton Rouge, LA 70809
(504) 926–6353

Maine
Health Care Review, Inc.
51 Broadway
Bangor, ME 04401
(207) 945–0244

Maryland
Delmarva Foundation for Medical Care,
 Inc.
341 North Aurora Street
Easton, MD 21601
(301) 822–0697

Massachusetts
Mass. Peer Review Organization, Inc.
300 Bearhill Road
Waltham, MA 02154
(617) 890–0011

Michigan
Michigan Peer Review Organization
40500 Ann Arbor Rd., Suite 200
Plymouth, MI 48170
(313) 459–0900

Minnesota
Foundation for Health Care Evaluation
One Appletree Square, Suite 700
Minneapolis, MN 55420
(612) 854–3306

Mississippi
Mississippi Foundation for Medical
 Care, Inc.

1900 North West St., P.O. Box 4665
Jackson, MS 39216
(601) 948–8894

Missouri
Missouri Patient Care Review
   Foundation
311 Ellis Blvd., Suite A
Jefferson City, MO 65101
(314) 634–4441

Montana
Montana-Wyoming Foundation for
   Medical Care
21 North Main, P.O. Box 5117
Helena, MT 59604
(406) 443–4020

Nebraska
Iowa Foundation for Medical Care (NE)
3737 Woodland Ave., Suite 500
West Des Moines, IA 50265
(515) 223–2900

Nevada
Nevada Physician Review Organization
Building A, Suite 108
4600 Kietzke Lane
Reno, NV 89502
(702) 826–1996

New Hampshire
New Hampshire Foundation for Medical
   Care
110 Locust St., P.O. Box 578
Dover, NH 03820
(603) 749–1641

New Jersey
Peer Review Organization of New
   Jersey, Inc., Central Division
Brier Hill Court, Bldg. J
East Brunswick, NJ 08816
(201) 238–5570

New Mexico
New Mexico Medical Review
   Association
Box Number 9900
Albuquerque, NM 87106
(505) 842–6236

New York
Empire State Medical Scientific and
   Educational Foundation, Inc.
420 Lakeview Road
Lake Success, NY 11042
(516) 437–8134

North Carolina
Medical Review of North Carolina, Inc.
1011 Schaub Dr., Suite 200
P.O. Box 37309
Raleigh, NC 27627
(919) 851–2955

North Dakota
North Dakota Health Care Review, Inc.
900 N. Broadway Ave., Suite 212
Minot, ND 58701
(701) 852–4231

Ohio
Peer Review Systems, Inc.
3700 Corporate Drive, Suite 250
Columbus, OH 43229
(614) 895–9900

Oklahoma
Oklahoma Foundation for Peer Review,
   Inc.
5801 Broadway Extension, Suite 400
Oklahoma City, OK 73118
(405) 840–2891

Oregon
Oregon Medical Professional Review
   Organization
1220 S.W. Morrison, Suite 300
Portland, OR 97205
(503) 243–1151

Pennsylvania
Keystone Peer Review Organization,
Inc.
645 North 12th St., P.O. Box 618
Lemoyne, PA 17043
(717) 975–9600

Rhode Island
Health Care Review, Inc.
The Weld Bldg., 345 Blackstone Blvd.
Providence, RI 02906
(401) 331–6661

South Carolina
Metrolina Medical Foundation
South Carolina PRO
3000 Charlottetown Center
Charlotte, NC 28204
(704) 373–1545

South Dakota
South Dakota Foundation for Medical
Care
1323 South Minnesota Avenue
Sioux Falls, SD 57105
(605) 336–3505

Tennessee
Mid-South Foundation for Medical Care
6401 Poplar Avenue, Suite 400
Memphis, TN 38119
(901) 682–0381

Texas
Texas Medical Foundation
Barton Oaks Plaza Two, Suite 200
901 Mopac Expressway South
Austin, TX 78746
(512) 329–6610

Utah
Utah Professional Standards Review
Organization
540 East 5th Street, South
Salt Lake City, UT 84102
(801) 532–7545

Vermont
New Hampshire Foundation for Medical
Care
110 Locust St., P.O. Box 578
Dover, NH 03820
(603) 749–1641

Virginia
Medical Society of Virginia Review
Organization
1904 Byrd Avenue, Room 120
Richmond, VA 23230
(804) 289–5320

Virgin Islands
Virgin Island Medical Institute
P.O. Box 1556, Christiansted
St. Croix, VI 00820
(809) 778–6470

Washington
Professional Review Organization for
Washington
2150 North 107th St., Suite 200
Seattle, WA 98133
(206) 364–9700

West Virginia
West Virginia Medical Institute, Inc.
3412 Chesterfield Ave., S.E.
Charleston, WV 25304
(304) 925–0461

Wisconsin
Wisconsin Peer Review Organization
2001 West Beltline Highway
Madison, WI 53713
(608) 274–1940

Wyoming
Montana-Wyoming Foundation for
Medical Care
21 North Main, P.O. Box 5117
Helena, MT 59604
(406) 443–4020

Appendix M

Medicare Part B Carriers

Alabama
Medicare Blue Cross–Blue Shield of
  Alabama
P.O. Box C–140
Birmingham, AL 35283
(205) 988–2244
(800) 292–8855

Alaska
Medicare, Aetna Life and Casualty
200 S.W. Market St., P.O. Box 1998
Portland, OR 97207
(503) 222–6831
(800) 547–6333

Arizona
Medicare, Aetna Life and Casualty
10000 N. 31st Ave., P.O. Box 37200
Phoenix, AZ 85069
(602) 861–1968
(800) 352–0411

Arkansas
Medicare, Arkansas Blue Cross and
  Blue Shield, a Mutual Insurance
  Company
P.O. Box 1418
Little Rock, AR 72203
(501) 378–2320
(800) 482–5525

California
*Counties of Los Angeles, Orange, San
  Diego, Ventura, Imperial, San Luis
  Obispo, Santa Barbara:*
Medicare, Transamerica Occidental Life
  Insurance Co.
Box 54905, Terminal Annex
Los Angeles, CA 90054
(213) 748–2311
(800) 252–9020

Rest of State:
Medicare Claims Department
Blue Shield of California
Chico, CA 95976
(714) 824–0900
(800) 952–8627 (Northern California)
(800) 848–7713 (Southern California)

Colorado
Medicare, Blue Shield of Colorado
700 Broadway
Denver, CO 80273
(303) 831–2661
(800) 332–6681

Connecticut
Medicare, The Travelers Insurance
  Company
100 Barnes Road North, P.O. Box 5005
Wallingford, CT 06493
(203) 728–6783
(800) 982–6819

Delaware
Medicare, Pennsylvania Blue Shield
P.O. Box 65
Camp Hill, PA 17011
(717) 763–3601
(800) 851–3535

District of Columbia
Medicare, Pennsylvania Blue Shield
P.O. Box 100
Camp Hill, PA 17011
(717) 763–3601
(800) 233–1124

Florida
Medicare, Blue Shield of Florida, Inc.
P.O. Box 2525
Jacksonville, FL 32231
(904) 355–3680
(800) 333–7586

Georgia
The Prudential Insurance Co. of
   America
Medicare Part B
P.O. Box 546
Buford, GA 30518
(404) 945–1401
(800) 241–3081

Hawaii
Medicare, Aetna Life and Casualty
P.O. Box 3947
Honolulu, HI 96812
(808) 524–1240
(800) 272–5242

Idaho
Medicare, EQUICOR, Inc.
P.O. Box 8048
Boise, ID 83707
(208) 342–7763
(800) 632–6574

Illinois
Blue Cross and Blue Shield of Illinois
Medicare Claims
P.O. Box 4422
Marion, IL 62959
(312) 938–8000
(800) 642–6930

Indiana
Medicare Claims, Part B, Associated
   Insurance Companies, Inc.
P.O. Box 7073
Indianapolis, IN 46207
(317) 842–4151
(800) 622–4792

Iowa
Medicare Claims, Blue Shield of Iowa
636 Grand Avenue
Des Moines, IA 50309
(515) 245–4785
(800) 532–1285

Kansas
Counties of Johnson, Wyandotte:
Medicare, Blue Shield of Kansas City
P.O. Box 169
Kansas City, MO 64141
(816) 561–0900
(800) 892–5900

Rest of State:
Medicare, Blue Shield of Kansas
P.O. Box 239
Topeka, KS 66601
(913) 232–3773
(800) 432–3531

Kentucky
Medicare Part B, Blue Cross/Blue
   Shield of Kentucky
100 East Vine Street
Lexington, KY 40507
(606) 233–1441
(800) 432–9255

Louisiana
Medicare, Blue Cross/Blue Shield of
 Louisiana
P.O. Box 95024
Baton Rouge, LA 70895
(504) 272–1242
(800) 462–9666

Maine
Medicare B, Blue Shield of
 Massachusetts/Tri-State
P.O. Box 1010
Biddeford, ME 04005
(207) 282–5991
(800) 492–0919

Maryland
*Counties of Montgomery, Prince
 Georges:*
Medicare, Pennsylvania Blue Shield
P.O. Box 100
Camp Hill, PA 17011
(717) 763–3601
(800) 233–1124

Rest of State:
Medicare, Blue Shield of Maryland, Inc.
700 East Joppa Road
Towson, MD 21204
(301) 561–4160
(800) 492–4795

Massachusetts
Medicare, Blue Shield of Massachusetts,
 Inc.
55 Accord Park Drive
Rockland, MA 02371
(617) 956–2126
(800) 882–1228

Michigan
Medicare Part B, Blue Cross/Blue
 Shield of Michigan
P.O. Box 2201
Detroit, MI 48231

(313) 225–8222
(800) 482–4045 (in area code 313)
(800) 322–0607 (in area code 517)
(800) 442–8020 (in area code 616)
(800) 562–7802 (in area code 906)

Minnesota
*Counties of Anoka, Dakota, Filmore,
 Goodhue, Hennepin, Houston,
 Olmstead, Ramsey, Wabasha,
 Washington, Winona:*
Medicare, The Travelers Insurance
 Company
8120 Penn Avenue, South
Bloomington, MN 55431
(612) 884–7171
(800) 352–2762

Rest of State:
Medicare, Blue Shield of Minnesota
P.O. Box 64357
St. Paul, MN 55164
(612) 456–5070
(800) 392–0343

Mississippi
Medicare, The Travelers Insurance
 Company
P.O. Box 22545
Jackson, MS 39225
(601) 956–0372
(800) 682–5417

Missouri
*Counties of Andrew, Atchison, Bates,
 Benton, Buchanan, Caldwell,
 Carroll, Cass, Clay, Clinton,
 Daviess, DeKalb, Gentry, Grundy,
 Harrison, Henry, Holt, Jackson,
 Johnson, Lafayette, Livingston,
 Mercer, Nodaway, Pettis, Platte,
 Ray, St. Clair, Saline, Vernon,
 Worth:*
Medicare, Blue Shield of Kansas City
P.O. Box 169

Kansas City, MO 64141
(816) 561–0900
(800) 892–5900

Rest of State:
Medicare, General American Life
  Insurance Company
P.O. Box 505
St. Louis, MO 63166
(314) 843–8880
(800) 392–3070

Montana
Medicare, Blue Shield of Montana
P.O. Box 4310
Helena, MT 59601
(406) 444–8350
(800) 633–1113

Nebraska
Medicare Claims, Blue Shield of Iowa
P.O. Box 10479
Des Moines, IA 50306
(402) 397–9182
(800) 633–1113

Nevada
Medicare, Aetna Life and Casualty
P.O. Box 37230
Phoenix, AZ 85069
(602) 861–1968
(800) 528–0311

New Hampshire
Medicare Part B, Blue Shield of
  Massachusetts/Tri-State
P.O. Box 1010
Biddeford, ME 04005
(207) 282–5991
(800) 447–1142

New Jersey
*Counties of Monmouth, Hunterdon,
  Somerset, Mercer, Ocean:*
Medicare, The Prudential Insurance Co.
  of America

P.O. Box 1000
Linwood, NJ 08221

*Counties of Camden, Atlantic, Cape
  May, Cumberland, Salem,
  Gloucester, Union, Middlesex: use
  same address as above except
  substitute:*
P.O. Box 2000

*Counties of Burlington, Morris, Warren,
  Sussex, Essex: use same address as
  above except substitute:*
P.O. Box 3333

*Counties of Passaic, Hudson, Bergen:
  use same address as above except
  substitute:*
P.O. Box 4000

Telephone numbers for all counties:
(609) 653–2700
(800) 462–9306

New Mexico
Medicare Claims/Administration, Aetna
  Life and Casualty of Oklahoma
P.O. Box 25500
Oklahoma City, OK 73125
(505) 843–7771
(800) 423–2925

New York:
*Counties and Boroughs of Bronx,
  Columbia, Delaware, Dutchess,
  Greene, Kings, Nassau, New York,
  Orange, Putnam, Richmond,
  Rockland, Suffolk, Sullivan, Ulster,
  Westchester:*
Medicare, Empire State Blue Cross/Blue
  Shield of New York
P.O. Box 4840, Grand Central Station
New York, NY 10163
(212) 490–4444
(800) 442–8430

Borough of Queens:
Medicare, Group Health, Inc.
P.O. Box A966, Times Square Station
New York, NY 10036
(212) 760–6790

Rest of State:
Medicare, Blue Shield of Western New
  York
P.O. Box 5200
Binghamton, NY 13902
(607) 772–6906
(800) 252–6550

North Carolina
The Prudential Insurance Co. of
  America, Medicare B Division
P.O. Box 2126
High Point, NC 27261
(919) 884–3400
(800) 672–3071

North Dakota
Medicare, Blue Shield of North Dakota
4510 13th Avenue, S.W.
Fargo, ND 58121
(701) 282–1100
(800) 247–2267

Ohio
Medicare, Nationwide Mutual Insurance
  Co.
P.O. Box 57
Columbus, OH 43216
(614) 249–7157
(800) 282–0530

Oklahoma
Medicare Administration, Aetna Life
  and Casualty
701 N.W. 63rd Street, Suite 300
Oklahoma City, OK 73116
(405) 848–7711
(800) 522–9079

Oregon
Medicare Administration, Aetna Life &
  Casualty
200 S.W. Market St., P.O. Box 1997
Portland, OR 97207
(503) 222–6831
(800) 452–0125

Pennsylvania
Medicare, Pennsylvania Blue Shield
Box 65, Blue Shield Building
Camp Hill, PA 17011
(717) 763–3601
(800) 382–1274

Puerto Rico
Medicare Part B, Seguros de Servicio de
  Salud de Puerto Rico
Call Box 71391
San Juan, PR 00936
(809) 759–9191
137 (800) 462–7385

Rhode Island
Medicare, Blue Shield of Rhode Island
444 Westminster Mall
Providence, RI 02901
(401) 861–2273
(800) 662–5170

South Carolina
Medicare, Blue Cross/Blue Shield of
  South Carolina
Fontaine Road Business Center
300 Arbor Lake Drive, Suite 1300
Columbia, SC 29223
(803) 754–0639
(800) 922–2340

South Dakota
Medicare, Blue Shield of North Dakota
4510 13th Avenue, S.W.
Fargo, ND 58121
(701) 282–0691
(800) 437–4762

Tennessee
Medicare, EQUICOR, Inc.
P.O. Box 1465
Nashville, TN 37202
(615) 244–5650
(800) 342–8900

Texas
Medicare, Blue Cross/Blue Shield of
    Texas, Inc.
P.O. Box 660031
Dallas, TX 75266
(214) 647–2282
(800) 442–2620

Utah
Medicare, Blue Shield of Utah
P.O. Box 30270, 2455 Parley's Way
Salt Lake City, UT 84130
(801) 481–6196
(800) 426–3477

Vermont
Medicare Part B, Blue Shield of
    Massachusetts/Tri-State
P.O. Box 1010
Biddeford, ME 04005
(207) 282–5991
(800) 447–1142

Virginia
*Counties of Arlington, Fairfax; Cities of
    Alexandria, Falls Church, Fairfax:*
Medicare, Pennsylvania Blue Shield
P.O. Box 100
Camp Hill, PA 17011
(717) 763–3601
(800) 233–1124

Rest of State:
Medicare, The Travelers Insurance Co.
P.O. Box 26463

Richmond, VA 23261
(804) 254–4130
(800) 552–3423

Virgin Islands
Serguros de Servicio de Salud de Puerto
    Rico
Call Box 71391
San Juan, PR 00936
(809) 759–9191
137 (800) 462–2970

Washington
Medicare, Washington Physicians'
    Service
4th and Battery Bldg., 6th Floor
2401 4th Avenue
Seattle, WA 98121
(206) 441–9370

West Virginia
Medicare, Nationwide Mutual Insurance
    Co.
P.O. Box 57
Columbus, OH 43216
(614) 249–7157
(800) 848–0106

Wisconsin
Medicare, Wisconsin Physicians'
    Service
Box 1787
Madison, WI 53701
(608) 221–3330
(800) 362–7221

Wyoming
Medicare, EQUICOR, Inc.
P.O. Box 628
Cheyenne, WY 82003
(307) 632–9381
(800) 442–2371

Appendix N

Medicaid Coverage of AIDS-Related Drugs

The following excerpt from Ben Schatz's *Access to AIDS-Related Drugs Under Medicaid: A Fifty-State Analysis* (San Francisco: National Gay Rights Advocates, 1989, $12.95; see appendix G–1 for ordering address; reprinted here by permission of National Gay Rights Advocates) contains a table setting forth coverage policies of the 50-odd state Medicaid programs for AIDS-related drugs, as of late 1988. The table should be used with care because (1) a few states indicated coverage of certain drugs, when, in fact, only inpatient and not outpatient coverage was offered; (2) FDA and NIH announcements and rulings, as well as continuing state policy changes, mean that state drug coverage will likely expand in subsequent months; and (3) the accompanying textual analysis in the full study is not reprinted here.

MEDICAID COVERAGE OF AIDS-RELATED DRUGS: RESULTS

STATE	GANCICLOVIR (DHPG) Yes	Some Cases	No		AZT (RETROVIR) Yes	Some Cases	No	ACYCLOVIR Yes	Some Cases	No		AEROSOLIZED PENTAMIDINE Yes	Some Cases	No	SEPTRA Yes	Some Cases	No	FANSIDAR Yes	Some Cases	No	DAPSONE Yes	Some Cases	No
ALABAMA			X	AIDS			X	X			AIDS, Previous PCP			X	X				X[1]			X[1]	
				ARC			X	X			AIDS, No Previous PCP			X	X				X[1]			X[1]	
				HIV+			X	X			ARC/HIV, No Previous PCP			X	X				X[1]			X[1]	
ALASKA			X	AIDS	X			X			AIDS, Previous PCP			X	X			X			X		
				ARC	X			X			AIDS, No Previous PCP			X	X			X			X		
				HIV+	X			X			ARC/HIV, No Previous PCP			X	X			X			X		
ARIZONA		X[11]		AIDS	X			X			AIDS, Previous PCP	X			X					X			X
				ARC		X		X			AIDS, No Previous PCP		X[11]			X[11]				X			X
				HIV+		X		X			ARC/HIV, No Previous PCP		X[11]			X[11]				X			X
ARKANSAS			X	AIDS		X[1]		X[5]			AIDS, Previous PCP	X[1]			X			X			X		
				ARC		X[1]		X[5]			AIDS, No Previous PCP	X[1]			X			X			X		
				HIV+		X[1]		X[5]			ARC/HIV, No Previous PCP	X[1]			X			X			X		
CALIFORNIA	X			AIDS		X[12]			X[13]		AIDS, Previous PCP	X[1]			X				X[1]			X[1]	
				ARC		X[12]			X[13]		AIDS, No Previous PCP		X[1]		X				X[1]			X[1]	
				HIV+		X[12]			X[13]		ARC/HIV, No Previous PCP		X[1]		X				X[1]			X[1]	
COLORADO	X[1]			AIDS			X[2]	X			AIDS, Previous PCP	X[1]			X			X[1]			X[1]		
				ARC			X[2]	X			AIDS, No Previous PCP	X[1]			X			X[1]			X[1]		
				HIV+			X[2]	X			ARC/HIV, No Previous PCP	X[1]			X			X[1]			X[1]		
CONNECTICUT	X			AIDS	X			X			AIDS, Previous PCP	X			X			X			X		
				ARC	X			X			AIDS, No Previous PCP	X			X			X			X		
				HIV+	X			X			ARC/HIV, No Previous PCP	X			X			X			X		
DELAWARE		X[14]		AIDS	X			X			AIDS, Previous PCP		X[14]		X			X			X		
				ARC	X			X			AIDS, No Previous PCP		X[14]		X			X			X		
				HIV+	X			X			ARC/HIV, No Previous PCP		X[14]		X			X			X		
FLORIDA			X	AIDS	X			X			AIDS, Previous PCP	X			X			X			X		
				ARC	X			X			AIDS, No Previous PCP	X			X			X			X		
				HIV+	X			X			ARC/HIV, No Previous PCP	X			X			X			X		
GEORGIA			X	AIDS	X[1]			X			AIDS, Previous PCP	X[1]			X			X[1]			X		
				ARC	X[1]			X			AIDS, No Previous PCP	X[1]			X			X[1]			X		
				HIV+	X[1]			X			ARC/HIV, No Previous PCP	X[1]			X			X[1]			X		
HAWAII			X	AIDS	X			X			AIDS, Previous PCP			X	X					X			
				ARC	X			X			AIDS, No Previous PCP			X		X				X			
				HIV+			X			X	ARC/HIV, No Previous PCP			X									X
IDAHO			X	AIDS	X			X			AIDS, Previous PCP	X			X			X			X		
				ARC	X			X			AIDS, No Previous PCP	X			X			X			X		
				HIV+	X			X			ARC/HIV, No Previous PCP	X			X			X			X		
ILLINOIS			X	AIDS	X			X			AIDS, Previous PCP		X[8]		X[9]			X			X		
				ARC	X			X			AIDS, No Previous PCP		X[8]		X[9]			X			X		
				HIV+	X			X			ARC/HIV, No Previous PCP		X[8]		X[9]			X			X		

MEDICAID COVERAGE OF AIDS-RELATED DRUGS: RESULTS

STATE		GANCICLOVIR (DHPG)			AZT (RETROVIR)			ACYCLOVIR				AEROSOLIZED PENTAMIDINE			SEPTRA			FANSIDAR			DAPSONE		
		Yes	Some Cases	No	Yes	Some Cases	No	Yes	Some Cases	No		Yes	Some Cases	No	Yes	Some Cases	No	Yes	Some Cases	No	Yes	Some Cases	No
INDIANA	AIDS				X			X			AIDS, Previous PCP	X			X			X			X		
	ARC			X	X			X			AIDS, No Previous PCP	X			X			X			X		
	HIV+				X			X			ARC/HIV, No Previous PCP	X			X								
IOWA	AIDS				X			X			AIDS, Previous PCP				X			X			X		
	ARC			X	X			X			AIDS, No Previous PCP			X	X			X			X		
	HIV+				X			X			ARC/HIV, No Previous PCP			X	X								
KANSAS	AIDS				X			X			AIDS, Previous PCP	X			X					X	X		
	ARC			X	X			X			AIDS, No Previous PCP	X			X					X	X		
	HIV+				X			X			ARC/HIV, No Previous PCP				X					X	X		
KENTUCKY	AIDS					X[1]			X[1]		AIDS, Previous PCP			X[6]	X			X[1]			X[1]		
	ARC			X		X[1]			X[1]		AIDS, No Previous PCP			X[6]	X			X[1]			X[1]		
	HIV+					X[1]			X[1]		ARC/HIV, No Previous PCP			X[6]	X			X[1]			X[1]		
LOUISIANA	AIDS				X			X			AIDS, Previous PCP			X[15]	X					X	X		
	ARC			X[15]	X			X			AIDS, No Previous PCP			X[15]	X					X	X		
	HIV+				X			X			ARC/HIV, No Previous PCP			X[15]	X					X	X		
MAINE	AIDS	X			X			X			AIDS, Previous PCP	X			X			X			X		
	ARC				X			X			AIDS, No Previous PCP	X			X			X			X		
	HIV+				X			X			ARC/HIV, No Previous PCP	X			X			X			X		
MARYLAND	AIDS				X			X			AIDS, Previous PCP	X			X			X			X[1]		
	ARC			X	X			X			AIDS, No Previous PCP	X			X			X			X[1]		
	HIV+				X			X			ARC/HIV, No Previous PCP	X			X			X			X[1]		
MASSACHUSETTS	AIDS				X			X			AIDS, Previous PCP	X[1]			X			X			X		
	ARC			X	X			X			AIDS, No Previous PCP			X	X			X			X		
	HIV+				X			X			ARC/HIV, No Previous PCP			X	X			X			X		
MICHIGAN	AIDS				X			X			AIDS, Previous PCP	X			X				X[16]		X		
	ARC		X[1]		X			X			AIDS, No Previous PCP			X	X				X[16]		X		
	HIV+				X			X			ARC/HIV, No Previous PCP			X	X				X[16]		X		
MINNESOTA	AIDS				X			X			AIDS, Previous PCP	X			X			X			X		
	ARC	X			X			X			AIDS, No Previous PCP	X			X			X			X		
	HIV+				X			X			ARC/HIV, No Previous PCP	X			X			X			X		
MISSISSIPPI	AIDS				X			X			AIDS, Previous PCP			X	X					X			X
	ARC			X			X	X			AIDS, No Previous PCP			X	X					X			X
	HIV+						X	X			ARC/HIV, No Previous PCP			X	X					X			X
MISSOURI	AIDS					X[1]			X		AIDS, Previous PCP		X[1]		X					X			X
	ARC		X			X[1]			X		AIDS, No Previous PCP			X	X					X			X
	HIV+					X[1]			X		ARC/HIV, No Previous PCP			X	X					X			X
MONTANA	AIDS				X			X			AIDS, Previous PCP	X			X			X			X		
	ARC			X	X			X			AIDS, No Previous PCP	X			X			X			X		
	HIV+				X			X			ARC/HIV, No Previous PCP	X			X			X					

PLEASE SEE PAGE 12 FOR CHART FOOTNOTES

MEDICAID COVERAGE OF AIDS-RELATED DRUGS: RESULTS

STATE		GANCICLOVIR (DHPG) Yes/Some	GANCICLOVIR No	AZT (RETROVIR) Yes/Some	AZT No	ACYCLOVIR Yes/Some	ACYCLOVIR No		AEROSOLIZED PENTAMIDINE Yes/Some	AEROSOLIZED PENTAMIDINE No	SEPTRA Yes/Some	SEPTRA No	FANSIDAR Yes/Some	FANSIDAR No	DAPSONE Yes/Some	DAPSONE No
NEBRASKA	AIDS		X	X		X		AIDS, Previous PCP		X	X		X		X	
	ARC			X		X		AIDS, No Previous PCP		X	X		X		X	
	HIV+			X		X		ARC/HIV, No Previous PCP		X	X		X			
NEVADA	AIDS		X	X		X		AIDS, Previous PCP		X	X		X			X
	ARC			X		X		AIDS, No Previous PCP		X[6]	X		X			X
	HIV+			X		X		ARC/HIV, No Previous PCP		X[6]	X		X			X
NEW HAMPSHIRE	AIDS		X	X		X		AIDS, Previous PCP	X		X		X		X	
	ARC			X		X		AIDS, No Previous PCP	X		X		X		X	
	HIV+			X		X		ARC/HIV, No Previous PCP	X		X		X		X	
NEW JERSEY	AIDS		X	X		X		AIDS, Previous PCP	X		X		X		X	
	ARC			X		X		AIDS, No Previous PCP	X		X		X		X	
	HIV+			X		X		ARC/HIV, No Previous PCP	X		X		X		X	
NEW MEXICO	AIDS	X		X		X		AIDS, Previous PCP	X		X		X		X	
	ARC			X		X		AIDS, No Previous PCP	X		X		X		X	
	HIV+			X		X		ARC/HIV, No Previous PCP	X		X		X		X	
NEW YORK	AIDS		X	X		X		AIDS, Previous PCP		X[6]	X		X		X	
	ARC			X		X		AIDS, No Previous PCP		X[6]	X		X		X	
	HIV+			X		X		ARC/HIV, No Previous PCP		X[6]	X		X		X	
NORTH CAROLINA	AIDS			X		X		AIDS, Previous PCP		X	X		X		X	
	ARC			X[3]		X		AIDS, No Previous PCP		X	X		X		X	
	HIV+			X[3]	X	X		ARC/HIV, No Previous PCP		X	X		X		X	
NORTH DAKOTA	AIDS		X	X		X		AIDS, Previous PCP	X		X[9]		X[1]		X	
	ARC			X		X		AIDS, No Previous PCP		X	X[9]		X[1]		X	
	HIV+				X		X	ARC/HIV, No Previous PCP		X	X[9]		X[1]		X	
OHIO	AIDS		X	X		X		AIDS, Previous PCP	X[8]		X		X		X	
	ARC			X		X		AIDS, No Previous PCP	X[8]		X		X		X	
	HIV+			X		X		ARC/HIV, No Previous PCP	X[8]		X		X		X	
OKLAHOMA	AIDS	X		X		X		AIDS, Previous PCP	X		X		X			X
	ARC			X		X		AIDS, No Previous PCP	X		X		X			X
	HIV+			X		X		ARC/HIV, No Previous PCP	X		X					X
OREGON	AIDS	X		X[4]		X		AIDS, Previous PCP	X[1]		X			X		X
	ARC			X[4]		X		AIDS, No Previous PCP	X		X			X		X
	HIV+				X	X		ARC/HIV, No Previous PCP		X	X					X
PENNSYLVANIA	AIDS		X	X		X		AIDS, Previous PCP		X	X		X		X	
	ARC			X		X		AIDS, No Previous PCP		X	X		X		X	
	HIV+			X		X		ARC/HIV, No Previous PCP		X	X		X		X	
RHODE ISLAND	AIDS	X		X		X		AIDS, Previous PCP	X		X		X		X	
	ARC			X		X		AIDS, No Previous PCP	X		X		X		X	
	HIV+			X		X		ARC/HIV, No Previous PCP	X		X		X		X	

MEDICAID COVERAGE OF AIDS-RELATED DRUGS: RESULTS

GANCICLOVIR (DHPG) / AZT (RETROVIR) / ACYCLOVIR

STATE	Category	GANCICLOVIR (DHPG) Yes	Some Cases	No	AZT (RETROVIR) Yes	Some Cases	No	ACYCLOVIR Yes	Some Cases	No
SOUTH CAROLINA	AIDS			X	X			X[10]		
	ARC				X			X[10]		
	HIV+				X			X[10]		
SOUTH DAKOTA	AIDS	X			X			X		
	ARC						X	X		
	HIV+						X	X		
TENNESSEE	AIDS			X	X			X		
	ARC				X			X		
	HIV+				X			X		
TEXAS	AIDS			X	X			X		
	ARC				X			X		
	HIV+						X	X		
UTAH	AIDS	X			X			X		
	ARC				X			X		
	HIV+					X[1]		X		
VERMONT	AIDS			X	X			X		
	ARC				X			X		
	HIV+				X			X		
VIRGINIA	AIDS			X	X			X[5]		
	ARC				X			X[5]		
	HIV+				X			X[5]		
WASHINGTON	AIDS			X	X			X		
	ARC					X		X		
	HIV+						X	X		
WEST VIRGINIA	AIDS			X	X[1]			X		
	ARC				X[1]			X		
	HIV+				X[1]			X		
WISCONSIN	AIDS			X	X			X		
	ARC				X			X		
	HIV+				X			X		
WYOMING	AIDS			X	X			X		
	ARC				X			X		
	HIV+				X			X		
DISTRICT OF COLUMBIA	AIDS			X	X			X		
	ARC				X			X		
	HIV+				X			X		
TOTAL	AIDS	11	4	36	45	4	2	49	2	0
	ARC				40	7	4	49	2	0
	HIV+				36	5	10	47	3	1

AEROSOLIZED PENTAMIDINE / SEPTRA / FANSIDAR / DAPSONE

STATE	Category	AEROSOLIZED PENTAMIDINE Yes	Some Cases	No	SEPTRA Yes	Some Cases	No	FANSIDAR Yes	Some Cases	No	DAPSONE Yes	Some Cases	No
SOUTH CAROLINA	AIDS, Previous PCP	X[1]			X[10]			X			X		
	AIDS, No Previous PCP			X	X[10]			X			X		
	ARC/HIV, No Previous PCP			X	X[10]			X			X		
SOUTH DAKOTA	AIDS, Previous PCP	X			X			X			X		
	AIDS, No Previous PCP	X			X			X			X		
	ARC/HIV, No Previous PCP	X			X			X			X		
TENNESSEE	AIDS, Previous PCP	X			X					X			X
	AIDS, No Previous PCP	X			X					X			X
	ARC/HIV, No Previous PCP	X			X					X			X
TEXAS	AIDS, Previous PCP			X	X					X			X
	AIDS, No Previous PCP			X	X					X			X
	ARC/HIV, No Previous PCP			X	X					X			X
UTAH	AIDS, Previous PCP	X			X			X			X		
	AIDS, No Previous PCP	X			X			X			X		
	ARC/HIV, No Previous PCP	X			X			X			X		
VERMONT	AIDS, Previous PCP	X			X			X			X		
	AIDS, No Previous PCP	X			X			X			X		
	ARC/HIV, No Previous PCP	X			X			X			X		
VIRGINIA	AIDS, Previous PCP			X[6,7]	X			X			X		
	AIDS, No Previous PCP			X[6,7]	X			X			X		
	ARC/HIV, No Previous PCP			X[6,7]	X			X			X		
WASHINGTON	AIDS, Previous PCP	X			X				X[11]			X[11]	
	AIDS, No Previous PCP			X	X				X[11]			X[11]	
	ARC/HIV, No Previous PCP			X	X				X[11]			X[11]	
WEST VIRGINIA	AIDS, Previous PCP	X[1]			X			X[1]			X[1]		
	AIDS, No Previous PCP	X[1]			X			X[1]			X[1]		
	ARC/HIV, No Previous PCP	X[1]			X			X[1]			X[1]		
WISCONSIN	AIDS, Previous PCP	X			X			X			X		
	AIDS, No Previous PCP	X			X			X			X		
	ARC/HIV, No Previous PCP	X			X			X			X		
WYOMING	AIDS, Previous PCP	X			X			X			X		
	AIDS, No Previous PCP	X			X			X			X		
	ARC/HIV, No Previous PCP	X			X			X			X		
DISTRICT OF COLUMBIA	AIDS, Previous PCP	X			X			X			X		
	AIDS, No Previous PCP	X			X			X			X		
	ARC/HIV, No Previous PCP	X			X			X			X		
TOTAL	AIDS, Previous PCP	33	4	14	51	0	0	37	5	9	41	3	7
	AIDS, No Previous PCP	26	5	20	50	1	0	37	5	9	41	3	7
	ARC/HIV, No Previous PCP	25	5	21	49	2	0	37	5	9	40	3	8

PLEASE SEE PAGE 12 FOR CHART FOOTNOTES

CHART FOOTNOTES

1   Prior authorization required.

2   Available only through federal grant—Medicaid merely administers (does not fund).

3   For adults only.

4   Provides if person meets FDA labeling indications.

5   Oral form of drug only.

6   Covers injectable pentamidine only.

7   Will cover when approved for marketing by FDA.

8   Officially pays only for injectable. However, unofficially, patient may obtain a nebulizer and injectable pentamidine.

9   Covers generic equivalent.

10   Prior authorization needed for home IV use.

11   Case-specific decision based on "medical necessity" or medical condition.

12   Prior authorization required if not used according to FDA labeling indications.

13   Prior authorization required except for herpes genitalis or for immunocompromised patients.

14   Not on Medicaid formulary, but may be payable as a compounded prescription. For hospitalized patients, may be included on pharmacy bill (non-itemized).

15   Under consideration for addition to formulary.

GLOSSARY

Terms In Report

AIDS
Acquired Immune Deficiency Syndrome. Most severe manifestation of HIV infection. Characterized by profound breakdown of the immune system accompanied by life-threatening opportunistic infections, wasting syndrome, and/or dementia.

ARC
AIDS-Related Complex. Middle spectrum of HIV disease, marked by weakened immune system and broad range of medical problems. Can be very severe, occasionally resulting in death.

FDA
U.S. Food and Drug Administration. The Federal agency responsible for approving and licensing drugs and medical devices.

HIV
Human Immunodeficiency Virus. The virus generally believed to cause AIDS and ARC by breaking down the immune system, leaving the body vulnerable to illness.

HIV+
Human Immunodeficiency Virus Positive. Unless otherwise indicated, this term is used in this report to indicate asymptomatic infection with HIV.

PCP
Pneumocystis carinii pneumonia. An opportunistic infection which is the most common cause of death in persons with AIDS.

PWA
Person with AIDS.

Treatment-IND
Treatment Investigational New Drug. Mechanism established by FDA to allow distribution of promising but unlicensed drugs to persons with life threatening conditions.

Drugs In Survey

Acyclovir
Capsules, ointment or powder. FDA labeling indicates use for genital herpes and herpes simplex. Also recommended by some physicians for use as an adjunct to AZT.

Aerosolized Pentamidine
At time of survey, only injectable (non-aerosolized) pentamidine was FDA approved for treatment of PCP. Aerosolized (inhalable) pentamidine was undergoing trials and not yet approved by the FDA. Nonetheless, the aerosolized form is widely believed by physicians to be safer and more effective both as a treatment and as a prophylaxis (preventative). Since the survey was conducted, aerosolized pentamidine was granted Treatment-IND status by the FDA.

AZT (Retrovir)
Oral medication. At time of survey, AZT was the only drug licensed specifically for treatment of AIDS and advanced cases of ARC. (Specifically for persons with PCP or T4 helper counts of less than 200.) It is widely being used for non-labeled uses to treat a broader range of HIV infection.

Dapsone
Oral medication. Licensed by FDA for treatment of leprosy. Recommended by some physicians for PCP.

Fansidar
Oral medication. FDA labeling indicates use for treatment/prevention of malaria. Recommended by some physicians for PCP.

Ganciclovir (DHPG)
Injectable drug. At time of survey, it was unlicensed but granted "compassionate use" status by the FDA for use against cytomegalovirus (CMV). ("Compassionate use" status allows manufacturers to release a drug free of charge on a case-by-case basis when no satisfactory

treatment exists.) Since the time of our survey, Ganciclovir has been granted Treatment-IND status.

Septra

Tablets or injectable. FDA labeling indicates use for treatment of urinary tract infections, chronic bronchitis, PCP and other illnesses.

Glossary

AARP: American Association of Retired Persons.

Acquired Immune Deficiency Syndrome (AIDS): A virus-caused fatal disease which destroys the human body's infection-fighting blood cells, leaving it defenseless against infections and cancers.

ACSW (Accredited Clinical Social Worker): Comparable to LCSW, where, in the absence or in lieu of state licensure, professional society accreditation permits the practice of clinical social work.

Administrative Law Judge (ALJ) hearing: SSA's counterpart, for its programs, to welfare agencies' fair hearings.

Adult day services: VA-sponsored day-long social service/care programs for incapacitated adults, on the model of senior citizens' day programs or children's day care centers.

Adult services: Social services such as counseling, home chore aid, meals-on-wheels, discharge planning, placement, abuse treatment, and so on, provided to adult welfare recipients as well as to some moderate-income aged and disabled people.

Aerosolized pentamidine: A medication sprayed through the mouth or nose into the lungs, which retards or prevents Pneumocystis carinii pneumonia (PCP), an often-fatal opportunistic infection common to PWAs.

AFDC (Aid to Families with Dependent Children): A federal-state welfare program for low-income families, commonly referred to as "welfare."

AFDC foster care: Foster care for children who originated in AFDC families, funded by federal-state AFDC program; includes Medicaid coverage of child.

AHCCCS (pronounced "Access"): Arizona Health Care Cost Containment System.

Aid and attendance: A VA term describing home chore aid which a disabled veteran pensioner must purchase because he is too incapacitated for daily living activities and for which he is therefore entitled to a higher pension income eligibility level.

Aid to the Permanently and Totally Disabled (APTD): A federal-state welfare program for poor disabled persons which was replaced by the federal SSI program in 1974; the phrase is still used in some states to refer to SSP programs.

AIDS: Acquired Immune Deficiency Syndrome.

Allowable charge: The total fee of a medical practitioner for a particular service which is recognized for payment purposes by Medicare (at 80%), Medicaid (at 100%), or private health insurance (at whatever percentage the plan specifies); not necessarily the same amount for these programs, since Medicaid's can be equal to or even lower than Medicare's, while health insurance plans recognize *far higher* amounts; determined in accordance with complex formulas specific to each program; also called "reasonable charge."

Alpha interferon: An anti-cancer medication useful in the treatment of PWAs, particularly for Kaposi's sarcoma, a carcinoma common to PWAs.

American Association of Retired Persons (AARP): A national membership organization of persons over the age of 50 which advocates for expanded public income and health programs.

Appeals council: SSA's in-house "supreme court" for further appeals of SSA program decisions from Administrative Law Judge hearings. Appeals almost always consist of a file review rather than an in-person hearing.

APTD: Aid to the Permanently and Totally Disabled.

ARC: AIDS-Related Complex.

Arizona Health Care Cost Containment System (AHCCCS): A health-care-for-the-poor program operated by Arizona with title XIX (Medicaid) funds.

Asset level: Asset amounts or values used in needs-based programs to determine eligibility for benefits; those with assets below the amount (or valued below the amount) are eligible, but those with assets above it are not.

Assets: Money and personal and real property owned by a benefits applicant.

Auxiliary grants: Generic state term for SSPs in Virginia.

Award letter: Letter or form from a government agency informing an applicant of approval for benefits and, if applicable, how much those benefits will be; SSDI, SSI, and VA notifications almost always state that disability is a basis for eligibility; AFDC, GA, Medicaid, and Food Stamps award letters may not explicitly state that incapacity or disability is a basis of eligibility, however (in which case those seeking proof of public disability benefits receipt should seek supplementary notes from their caseworkers).

AZT (zidovudine): Known also by the trade name Retrovir, a drug developed and marketed by Burroughs-Wellcome Pharmaceuticals—the only drug known (as of mid-1989) to retard the replication of the HIV virus.

Bad debt: Unpaid hospital bills, including—in some hospitals' usages—in-house charity care, Hill-Burton cases, and balances where the hospital "charges" more than Medicare, Medicaid, and insurance contracts allow; also, of course, ordinary delinquent accounts.

Board and care home: A publicly or privately operated residence which provides personal assistance, lodging, and meals to two or more adults unrelated to the operator. Also called custodial, domiciliary, personal care, adult foster, congregate, old age, community, and rest homes. Rents are paid with residents' private income and—for the needy—SSI and SSPs.

Buy-in: Procedure, effectively mandatory since 1969, whereby state Medicaid programs pay Part B Medicare premiums for those eligible for both programs; by extension, sometimes meant to describe the pre-1989 practice whereby states paid

Medicare deductibles and coinsurance, as well as premiums, for those on both programs; see Qualified Medicare Buy-In for the newly expanded, mandatory buy-in provision.

Categorically needy: In Medicaid parlance, those who receive Medicaid because they receive, are eligible for, or are *deemed* eligible for, AFDC, SSI, or SSPs.

Charity care coordinator: Financial counselor.

Child and family services: Social services provided to children and their parents, such as counseling, home chore aid, child-rearing and housekeeping training, and abuse treatment; especially for welfare recipients, but sometimes provided to other modest-income families.

COBRA: Consolidated Omnibus Budget Reconciliation Act of 1985.

Coinsurance: The percentage of allowable charges for a given class of medical care which the patient is left to pay, in Medicare and health insurance plans (for example, 20% of doctor's allowable charges under Medicare).

Community residence home care: The VA's term for board and care home services.

Compensation: Income payments the VA makes to veterans injured or who become ill while on active duty.

Conditional eligibility: The procedure to grant temporary SSI benefits to applicants with slightly too much in assets while they attempt to sell them and then repay program payments out of proceeds; by extension, this term is sometimes applied to situations where an applicant is granted eligibility even though he has excess assets (such as rural property for which there is no market) in both the SSI and Medicaid programs.

Consolidated Omnibus Budget Reconciliation Act of 1985 (COBRA): The federal law which, among other things, required employers of 20 or more to permit continued enrollment of ex-employees in group health insurance plans; when "COBRA" is mentioned, it almost always refers to this provision.

Copayment: Strictly speaking, a defined monetary amount a patient pays for a health service, with his or her health plan covering remaining costs (for example, $74.00 for last 80 days of SNF care under Medicare, 50¢ per prescription in many Medicaid programs); however, also used, by extension, synonymously with "coinsurance."

Cost share: Term used in California, Hawaii and other states for "spend down."

Countable income: The amount of income which needs-based programs compare to their income levels to determine eligibility, after disregarding specified amounts or percentages of gross income.

County relief: General assistance (GA).

Coupon/Food Stamp coupons: Forms issued by the U.S. Department of Agriculture which look somewhat like *Monopoly* money and which recipients use as money to purchase food at grocery stores.

Date of onset: The date on which an SSDI, SSI, or Medicaid applicant first became disabled within the meaning of the Social Security Act; almost always before the application, first treatment, or even work-cessation date.

DD214: Military discharge certificate which all veterans must present when applying for VA services.

Deductible: The amount of medical bills which a patient must incur before Medicare or health insurance coverage begins, usually on an annual basis; also, term traditionally used for "spend down" in North Carolina.

"Deeming" income and assets: The procedure, in eligibility determinations by needs-based programs, of lumping together the income of separate nuclear family members (even if they claim not to be sharing income) who live together in common households; for example, the incomes of spouses, or parent and child, living together, are combined (even over their objections) and compared to a two-person eligibility level, rather than to two separate one-person levels; the welfare system's version of the old adage, "two can live as cheaply as one."

Department of Health and Human Services (HHS): The federal agency responsible for almost all health and welfare programs; includes HCFA, PHS, and SSA.

Department of Housing and Urban Development (HUD): The federal agency which operates the public housing, rent supplement, low-income housing assistance, and FHA and HUD mortgage insurance programs.

Department of Veterans Affairs (VA): A federal agency which operates a variety of income and medical care programs for certain disabled veterans, some other veterans and, in some cases, their dependents.

Disability: A medical condition preventing work; under the Social Security Act, a medical condition lasting 12 or more months, or which will result in death, and which prevents any substantial gainful activity (earnings).

Disregards of assets: Amounts, values, or percentages of an applicant's assets which needs-based programs do not count in determining eligibility for benefits.

Disregards of income: Amounts or percentages of an applicant's gross income which needs-based programs do not count in determining eligibility for benefits.

EA: Emergency Assistance.

Emergency Assistance (EA): A federal-state welfare program which makes one-time crisis payments to or on behalf of low-income families with children and—in many states—the poor aged and disabled.

Exempt assets: Assets which are not considered or counted at all in determining benefit eligibility, such as lived-in homes under the SSI and VA pension programs.

Extended period of eligibility: 15 months of continued SGA work by an SSDI recipient, after the "trial work period," during which (1) SSDI checks stop after 3 months; (2) Medicare continues; but (3) during which an ex-SSDI recipient who ceases SGA can regain SSDI without a full-dress application.

Fair hearing: A semi-judicial proceeding before a state welfare officer at which an applicant or recipient for almost all state-administered benefits can present claims of error, unfairness, misapplication of rules, etc. to attempt a reversal or modification of an unfavorable decision on his case.

FDA: Food and Drug Administration.

Financial counselor: Hospital employee who assists indigents in applying for
Medicaid, Hill-Burton, GMA, or in-house charity care.

Food and Drug Administration (FDA): An arm of HHS's Public Health Service
which approves and licenses drugs for medical use.

Food and Nutrition Service (FNS): An agency within the U.S. Department of
Agriculture which administers the Food Stamp and Women, Infants, and Children
(WIC) programs.

Food Stamp program: A federally financed, state-run welfare program which gives
low-income persons vouchers with which to purchase food.

Foster care: Placement of an orphaned, abandoned, abused, or neglected child with
an adult or facility which provides the care the child's parents cannot; supervised
by welfare office caseworkers.

FS: Food Stamp program.

Future Medicare eligibility date: Two years after first eligibility for SSDI benefits.

GA: General Assistance.

General Assistance (GA): A generic term used for state-local welfare programs for
poor persons who are not coverable by the federal SSI and AFDC programs.

General Medical Assistance (GMA): State and local programs to provide health care
to poor persons who are not coverable by the federal Medicaid program.

General Relief (GR): General Assistance (GA), especially in New England and North
Central states.

GMA: General Medical Assistance.

Hill-Burton: A health facility grant and loan program, operated by the Health
Resources and Services Administration (HRSA) in HHS's Public Health Service;
beneficiary facilities must give specified amounts of free care to poor persons and
assure important health care access rights to area residents.

HIV (human immunodeficiency virus): The agent which causes AIDS; also used
generically to denote the full progressive spectrum of disease states culminating in
AIDS—HIV-positive, then "ARC," and finally "full-blown AIDS."

Home and community-based services: Under Medicaid's 2176 waiver program, these
are home health care, home chore aid, personal attendant, outpatient hospice,
visiting nurse, and even board and care home services which are offered as an
alternative to more expensive hospitalization or nursing home care.

Home health services: Health services given to a patient in his own home which can
be provided only by a licensed professional such as a registered nurse or physical,
speech or occupational therapist, and which can include unskilled care such as
housekeeping, feeding, and grooming assistance only when it is supportive to the
core health service which only the licensed professional can render. Covered by
Medicare, Medicaid, and many private health insurances.

Home relief (HR): Generic term for GA, and sometimes AFDC, in New York.

Hospice: A medical facility primarily engaged in providing care, including nursing,
physician, and palliative services, to terminally ill patients—at the facility, at the

patient's home, or both. Covered by Medicare, Medicaid, and some private health insurances.

Housebound: A VA term describing disabled veteran pensioners who are so incapacitated that they cannot leave their homes, medical facilities, or community residences without assistance and who are therefore entitled to a higher pension income eligibility level; sometimes used in the Medicaid and social services programs for vendor payment purchases of these services.

HUD: The federal Department of Housing and Urban Development.

HUD voucher: Documents of various denominations given to qualified low-income persons which they present to participating landlords for rent payment; landlords, in turn, redeem them for cash from HUD; a housing program counterpart to Food Stamps.

Impairment: A particular disease or condition afflicting a patient which may, in SSA parlance, render him too disabled to perform substantial gainful activity (SGA) and thus possibly eligible; patients can and do have multiple impairments.

Incapacity/Incapacitated parent: A disability, which can be lesser or less long-lasting than that required for SSDI/SSI, used to qualify a parent and thus (even in a two-parent family) a whole low-income family, for AFDC and Medicaid; sometimes used in GA programs too.

Income level: Income amounts used in needs-based programs, usually on a monthly basis, to determine eligibility for benefits; those with income below the level are eligible but those with income above it are not.

Income maintenance: Generic term for welfare, including GA, AFDC, and SSPs; used in New York and several other states.

Indigent: A poor person—and especially in a hospital context—a poor person without health care coverage.

Indigent care coordinator: Financial counselor.

Indigent care program: State, local (GMA), or hospital free medical care program for the poor; increasingly used for public subsidies or rate allowances to compensate hospitals for bad debts of indigents, rather than for a recipient-entitled-oriented program.

Intermediate care facility (ICF): A facility which provides health-related care and services to individuals who do not require the degree of care and treatment SNFs provide; the bulk of nursing home patients need ICF- rather than SNF-level care; Medicaid and cash payments are the sole sources of financing this level of care—it is not covered by Medicare or health insurance.

LCSW (Licensed Clinical Social Worker): A holder of the MSW degree who has been licensed by the state to practice psychiatric social work therapy.

Legal Aid Societies: Local philanthropic organizations which provide free legal services for the poor.

Legal Services Corporation: A federal instrument which funds neighborhood legal services for the poor across the country and supports national issue-specific legal think tanks.

LIHEA: The Low Income Home Energy Assistance program.

Listing of Impairments: A comprehensive listing, in SSDI and SSI regulations, of the most common diseases and medical conditions, including standards of diagnosis, medical proof, and evaluation to determine disability.

Lived-in home: A residence owned and actually dwelled in by an applicant for or recipient of assistance; generally, the only kind of real estate permitted by welfare programs.

Long-term care: Generic phrase describing care, usually of over 30 days, in mental hospitals, specialized rehabilitative hospitals, skilled nursing facilities, intermediate care facilities, board and care homes, and sometimes, hospices.

Low Income Home Energy Assistance (LIHEA): A federally funded program, operated by HHS, to pay heating, air conditioning, and home weatherization costs for low-income people.

LSC: Legal Services Corporation.

MA: Medical assistance.

Medicaid: A federal-state medical assistance program for certain kinds of poor people; operated by state health or welfare agencies under rules of the Health Care Financing Administration (HCFA) in the U.S. Department of Health and Human Services (HHS).

Medi-Cal: California's name for its Medicaid program.

Medical assistance (MA): A generic term to denote Medicaid, General Medical Assistance (GMA), and other health care programs for the poor.

Medically needy: In Medicaid parlance, persons who share characteristics with AFDC or SSI recipients, but who have incomes above AFDC, SSI, or SSI/SSP eligibility levels; at state option, medically needy people can receive Medicaid when their income is below (or, through "spend down," when it falls below) a state-set medically needy income level set anywhere between the AFDC level and an amount one-third higher.

Medicare: A health insurance program for those over age 65 or disabled, operated by the Health Care Financing Administration (HCFA) in the U.S. Department of Health and Human Services (HHS).

MSW: Master of Social Work, a graduate academic degree required for many professional-level welfare and hospital social work positions.

Municipal aid: General assistance (GA), especially in New Jersey.

NAN: National AIDS Network.

NAPWA: National Association of People With AIDS.

National AIDS Network (NAN): A national association of local groups providing advocacy, social work, and health-related services to people with HIV disease.

National Association of People With AIDS (NAPWA): An advocacy and self-help organization for people with HIV disease.

National Institutes of Health: An arm of HHS's Public Health Service that conducts medical research programs, which in many cases entail actual patient treatment.

Neighborhood legal services: Generic name for local law offices serving the poor for free; funded by the federal Legal Services Corporation (LSC).

NIH: National Institutes of Health.

Non-AFDC foster care: Foster care for children who did not originate in AFDC families, funded by state and local welfare programs; usually includes Medicaid coverage of child.

OASDI (Old Age, Survivors, and Disability Insurance): Formerly used to refer collectively to the range of worker-based income insurance programs operated by SSA for the insured aged, disabled, and their families.

Opportunistic infection: Diseases borne by viruses and bacteria which are ordinarily present in the environment and which are almost always fought off by the body, but which infect, sicken, and eventually kill those with compromised immune systems (such as persons with AIDS).

Part A: Medicare's hospital insurance, which covers basic room and board, inpatient drugs, operating room, recovery room, intensive care, hospices, home health care, and skilled nursing facility care; generally, has no premium for patients.

Part B: Medicare's medical insurance, which covers doctor bills, emergency rooms, hospital outpatient services, ambulances, certain inpatient hospital "extras," and home health care; patients must pay a premium for coverage.

Participation: Term traditionally used in Washington state for "spend down."

Patient pay: Term used in a number of states for "spend down," especially for nursing home patients.

Pension: Generic term for any public or employer retirement or disability income benefit; VA income program for needy veterans; euphemism for welfare grants, especially SSPs, in Alabama.

Personal needs allowance: The amount ($30, sometimes more) which a long-term hospital patient and nursing home and board and care residents are permitted to retain for "spending money," with the balance of their incomes applied to cost of care; by extension, the $30 monthly SSI benefit paid to institutionalized Medicaid patients with no other income.

PHS: Public Health Service.

Poverty level: A national income amount promulgated annually by the U.S. Department of Health and Human Services (HHS), which denotes the minimal amount necessary for basic living costs; used for Medicaid, Hill-Burton, and other needs-based programs. In 1990, it was about $522 monthly for a single individual.

Premium: Amount paid periodically by an insured person or employer to secure health insurance coverage from Medicare or a private health plan; also used for payments to maintain life insurance.

Presumptive disability determination: The procedure whereby Social Security district offices can find needy applicants with selected impairments (usually fairly obvious ones) to be disabled so that they can immediately begin receiving SSI payments; thus, pressing living expenses and medical care (through Medicaid) needs of desperate, newly disabled persons can be met while a full-dress disability determination of the medical records is conducted; up to 3 months of SSI checks can be paid under this provision. Since February 9, 1988, full-blown AIDS (but not ARC) diagnoses can allow for presumptive disability determinations.

PROs (Peer Review Organizations): Nonprofit organizations, usually arms of state medical societies, which review the appropriateness of care and lengths of stay under Medicaid and Medicare.

Public aid: Generic term for welfare in some states; used in Illinois for GA, AFDC, and even SSPs.

Public assistance (PA): Generic term for welfare, especially GA and AFDC; used in Maryland, the District of Columbia, and several other states.

Public Health Service (PHS): A U.S. agency within the Department of Health and Human Services (HHS) which operates the AZT assistance, AIDS education and prevention, low-income clinic, Hill-Burton, and Indian Health Service programs.

Public Law 92–603: The 1972 federal statute which created SSI; abolished the old state welfare programs for the aged, blind, and disabled; extended Medicare to the disabled; authorized State Supplementary Payments (SSPs); and offered states a set of complex options in coordinating SSI, SSP, and Medicaid eligibility.

PWA: Person with AIDS.

PWARC: Person with AIDS-related complex, once called "pre-AIDS."

QMB: Qualified Medicare Buy-In.

Qualified Medicare Buy-In (QMB) patient: An aged or disabled Medicare patient with income below the poverty level for whom the state Medicaid program must pay Medicare premiums, deductibles, and coinsurance.

Reasonable charge: Allowable charges, especially in Medicare and Medicaid.

Reconsideration: For SSA programs, a second determination of eligibility or related issues by a different worker, which may be requested by dissatisfied applicants or recipients.

Recoupment: Deducting the amount of past overpayments from ongoing or future benefit payments, usually in installments; used by the VA, SSDI, SSI, and welfare programs.

Redemption centers: Welfare offices, banks, and inner-city, storefront check-cashing facilities where Food Stamp recipients or their designees present monthly authorization forms for actual issuance of Food Stamp coupons.

Residual Functional Capacity (RFC): In SSA disability determinations, where a patient's medical condition(s) does not explicitly appear in, or clearly equal, maladies in SSA's *Listing of Impairments,* the RFC is used as a medical assessment of a person's work setting abilities in spite of his or her functional limitations and environmental restrictions imposed by all of his or her medically determinable impairments, such as the capacity for sustained performance of physical and mental job requirements. The RFC method, rather than the *Listing,* must always be used for "ARC-only" claimants; it is also sometimes relied upon for full-blown AIDS cases, as AIDS has not historically appeared in the *Listing.*

Resources: Welfare "bureaucratese" for assets.

Retroactive Medicaid eligibility date: The date, up to the first of the 3 full months prior to the month of application, back to which an applicant can later be found eligible if *at that time also,* he met income, asset, and disability rules.

Retrovir: AZT.

RFC: Residual Functional Capacity.

Section 1619 of the Social Security Act: Allows for continued payment of SSI benefits to working disabled recipients, without regard to the SGA, trial work period, and extended-period-of-eligibility limitations imposed by the companion SSDI program; allows disabled workers whose earnings raise them over the SSI income eligibility level to continue to be deemed to be SSI recipients for purposes of Medicaid coverage if the Medicaid-purchased care is what has been and is enabling them to "work their way off welfare" and if they cannot otherwise secure such medical care.

SF–180: Standard Form 180, Request Pertaining to Military Records.

SGA: Substantial Gainful Activity.

1616 states: States which arrange to have their SSPs paid out by the Social Security Administration (SSA) on top of, and as part of, the basic federal SSI payment; they reimburse SSA for these SSPs.

1634 states: States which automatically grant Medicaid to SSI recipients under contract arrangements with the Social Security Administration.

Skilled nursing facility (SNF): A facility which provides skilled nursing (such as that given by R.N.s) and related services for patients requiring the most intense and professional nursing home care; also called extended care; covered by Medicare, Medicaid, and some private health insurance.

Social Security Administration (SSA): An agency within the U.S. Department of Health and Human Services (HHS) which operates the SSDI and SSI programs and determines eligibility for Medicare and (in some cases) Medicaid.

Social Security Disability Insurance (SSDI): A federal income insurance program, operated by the Social Security Administration (SSA), for workers whom it determines are disabled.

Social Services Block Grant (SSBG): A federal program, administered by the U.S. Department of Health and Human Services (HHS), which authorizes grants to states for social services to the needy; replaced the former Title XX program, but often still called "Title XX."

Spend down: The process by which a Medicaid applicant with income above the eligibility level can deduct incurred medical bills from income so as to reduce it to the eligibility level and thereby secure coverage.

SSA: Social Security Administration.

SSDI: Social Security Disability Insurance.

SSI: Supplemental Security Income.

SSI/SSP: The combined, total SSI and SSP income/eligibility level for poor aged and disabled people for a given state or living arrangement.

SSP: State Supplementary Payment.

Standard Form 180, Request Pertaining to Military Records (SF–180): Federal form, available at VA offices, which a VA disability compensation applicant completes to obtain his military medical and personnel records for submission with his VA claim.

State Supplementary Payment (SSP): State welfare payments added to the basic federal SSI level, thereby raising the income minimum for poor aged, blind, and disabled people.

Subsidized employment: Where an employee does not fully "earn his own way" and where his paycheck is actually partial or full "disguised charity"; used by Social Security for handicapped workshops and the like, where earnings are not fully genuine (but are nonetheless paid) for charitable, morale, or therapeutic reasons; by extension, applied to situations where a no-longer-productive, deteriorating worker is continued on the payroll for altruistic purposes.

Substantial Gainful Activity (SGA): SSA term; work earnings over $300 monthly, which render otherwise disabled persons ineligible for SSDI.

Supplemental Security Income (SSI): A federal welfare program, operated by the Social Security Administration (SSA) with general revenues, which makes monthly payments to poor aged, blind, and disabled people.

TEFA: Temporary Emergency Food Assistance.

Temporary Emergency Food Assistance (TEFA): A federal program to distribute surplus federal food to needy people.

Title II: The Old Age, Survivors, and Disability Insurance section of the Social Security Act.

Title IV–A: The AFDC section of the Social Security Act.

Title VI and Title XVI of the Public Health Service Act: Sections which authorize and set forth the requirements of the federal Hill-Burton program.

Title XIV: The APTD (Aid to the Permanently and Totally Disabled) section of the Social Security Act.

Title XVI: The SSI section of the Social Security Act.

Title XVI state: A state which gives Medicaid to all SSI recipients, but not automatically—it requires aged, blind, and disabled applicants to apply separately for Medicaid at the welfare office, bringing proof of SSI eligibility.

Title XVIII: The Medicare section of the Social Security Act.

Title XIX: The Medicaid section of the Social Security Act.

Title XX: The section of the Social Security Act which provided grants to states for social services to the needy; since replaced by the Social Services Block Grant (SSBG) program, which itself continues to be referred to often as "Title XX."

Trial work period: Up to 9 months during which an SSDI recipient is permitted to earn over the monthly SGA level of $300, yet retain SSDI benefits and Medicare; originally designed as an incentive for attempts at recovery/return to work for the disabled, who would not lose benefits if their poor health undermined the work attempt.

2176 waivers: Exemptions from Medicaid rules and laws, authorized by the Health

Care Financing Administration (HCFA), which allow states to offer some or all disabled or aged people a wider array of home and community-based services—as alternatives to institutionalization—than is ordinarily available through Medicaid; these can include liberalized eligibility standards.

209(b) states: States which have retained some or all pre-SSI eligibility rules for the aged, blind, and disabled. Consequently, these people cannot get Medicaid automatically through SSI receipt but must apply for Medicaid under the stricter rules at the welfare office.

Unemployed parent: In the AFDC (Aid to Families with Dependent Children) program, the highest-earning parent, now unemployed over 30 days, whose unemployment qualifies even a two-parent family for AFDC and Medicaid, if they are also poor enough.

VA: Department of Veterans Affairs.

Verification: The means by which an applicant for benefits, or sometimes the eligibility worker, proves his allegations as to citizenship, residency, age, disability and poverty (see appendix E).

Veterans Outreach Centers: VA "storefront"-style offices, in many neighborhoods across the country, where veterans receive counseling, group therapy, substance abuse referrals, and assistance in applying for VA benefits.

Waiver: The procedure by which rules of the Social Security Act programs can be set aside by the Department of Health and Human Services (HHS), usually for experimental, research, or demonstration project purposes.

Welfare: Generic term for needs-based benefit programs for the needy, especially income programs; used by the lay public to refer to AFDC and sometimes GA.

WIC: Women, Infants, and Children program.

Women, Infants, and Children (WIC): A federally funded, state-run program to provide supplementary food and health-related assistance to pregnant women, nursing mothers, and children under age 5; operated at the federal level by the Food and Nutrition Service, WIC operates through local health departments, low-income health clinics, and sometimes welfare offices.

Zidovudine: AZT.

Annotated Bibliography

(See appendix G–1 for addresses and telephone numbers to order these publications.)

*Recommended reading.

**Particularly recommended for those doing intense/high volume benefits advocacy for PWAs and PWARCs.

Access to Health Care in the United States: Results of a 1986 Survey. Princeton: Robert Wood Johnson Foundation, 1986.

American Association of Retired Persons. *The AARP Guide to State Energy Assistance Offices.* Washington, D.C.: AARP, 1986. Free.

*American Association of Retired Persons. *A Checklist of Concerns/Resources for Caregivers* and *Miles Away and Still Caring.* Washington, D.C.: AARP, 1987. Free. Essential for local AIDS social services, buddy, and significant other support programs. Offers good referrals and bibliography.

American Association of Retired Persons. *Federal and State Legislative Policy, 1989.* Washington, D.C.: AARP, 1989. Free.

**Anders, S. *Health Care News* (periodical). Washington, D.C.: National Health Care Campaign, 1987–. $10.00/year. General advocacy for improved Medicaid, Medicare, and indigent health programs.

Andrulis, D. "State Medicaid Policies and Hospital Care for AIDS Patients" in *Health Affairs* 5(Winter 1987): 110.

Andrulis, D., *et al.* "The Provision and Financing of Medical Care for AIDS Patients in U.S. Public and Private Teaching Hospitals" in *Journal of the American Medical Association* 258 (1987): 1343.

Bartlett, L., and J. Hoffman. *State Options for Improving Access to Care for the Uninsured.* Washington, DC: Health System Research, Inc., 1987.

**Beyer, G., I. Bulkley, and P. Hopkins. "A Model Act Regulating Board and Care Homes: Guidelines for States" in *Mental and Physical Disability Law Reports* 8 (1984): 150. (Also available with related materials from AARP). Basic standards for the kinds of group homes many PWAs need.

**Bonnyman, G., and A. Robertson. "Making the Medicaid Spend Down Program Work: A Partnership of Community Education and Administrative Advocacy" in *Clearinghouse Review* 18(June 1987): 105. Chicago: National Clearinghouse for Legal Services. $6.00. How to run and use a "medically needy spend down" in state Medicaid programs.

*Brown, R., ed. *The Rights of Older Persons*. Carbondale: Southern Illinois University Press, 1989. $9.45. Good "layman's" question and answer treatment of SSDI, SSI, Medicaid, Medicare, and other programs, but still somewhat "lawyerly" and nonspecific on actual eligibility practice.

*Buchanan, R. "State Medicaid Coverage of AZT and AIDS-Related Policies" in *American Journal of Public Health,* April, 1988. AZT, prescriptions, waivers, and hospice coverage in state Medicaid programs.

Butler, D. *Health Care Financing Review. 1985 Supplement: 20 Years of Medicare and Medicaid.* Baltimore: HCFA, 1985.

*Butler, P. *Too Poor To Be Sick.* Washington, DC: American Public Health Assoc., 1988. $17.50. The A-to-Z story about state Medicaid and indigent health care programs today.

Carbine, M., and P. Lee. *AIDS Into the 90's: Strategies for an Integrated Response to the AIDS Epidemic.* Washington, DC: National AIDS Network, 1988. Free to members.

Carlson, J. *Health Care Campaign Guide.* Washington, DC: AARP, 1988. Free. How to organize to reform health care locally.

**Capitman, J. "Present and Future Roles of SSI and Medicaid in Funding Board and Care Homes" in M. Moon, G. Gaberlavage, and S. Newman, eds. *Preserving Independence, Supporting Needs: The Role of Board and Care Homes.* Washington, DC: AARP, 1989. Free.

*Carter, Nicala. *Resources for Nonlawyers.* Chicago: National Clearinghouse for Legal Services, 1985. Free. Good bibliography on social work and entitlements advocacy for non-attorney benefits advocates.

**Carty, Lee, ed. *Federal and State Rights and Entitlements for People Who Are Homeless.* Washington, DC: Mental Health Law Project, 1988. $20.00. Generic national manual, but "customized" editions available for at least 6 states, in a comprehensive format similar to that of *AIDS Benefits Handbook.* However, discussion is tailored to poverty lawyers and others already well versed in welfare.

*Center for Social Welfare Policy and the Law. *Reference and Statistical Sources for Legal Research in Public Assistance Programs.* Chicago: National Clearinghouse for Legal Services, 1987. Free. Order no. 30,211C. Excellent bibliography.

*Charleston-Pinnola, C., and H. Jordan. *Veterans Administration Programs for Disabled Veterans: An Overview.* Chicago: National Clearinghouse for Legal Services, 1986. $2.50. Order no. 40,900.

**Chen, A. "Board and Care Homes: The Cost of Operation" in M. Moon, G. Gaberlavage, and S. Newman, eds. *Preserving Independence, Supporting Needs: The Role of Board and Care Homes.* Washington, DC: AARP, 1989. Free.

Chollert, D. *Uninsured in the United States: The Nonelderly Population Without Health Insurance.* Washington, DC: The Employee Benefit Research Institute, 1987.

*Christ, Linda. *Social Security Disability Training Manual.* Chicago: National Clearinghouse for Legal Services, 1986. $35.00. Order no. 41,875.

Clinton, J. *AIDS Funding*. New York: The Foundation Center, 1988. $35.00. Where AIDS organizations can seek grants.

Cohen, J., and J. Holahan. *Medicaid: The Trade Off Between Cost Containment and Access to Care*. Washington, DC: Urban Institute, 1987. $12.95.

**Cohen, R., and M. Haske. *A Home Away From Home*. Washington, DC: AARP, 1986. Free. A superb introduction to Board and Care Home programs; the appendixes—especially the bibliography—are invaluable.

**Coopers and Lybrand, Inc. *An Addendum to the Model Act: Financial Incentives For Board and Care Facilities*. Washington, DC: American Bar Association Rights of the Aged Project, 1984. $7.50. Difficult to read, this is still the basic text on how to finance startup and operation of a board and care home (language and format are for accountants, lawyers, and real estate developers rather than for small community nonprofit groups—moreover, some programs or financing schemes are being rapidly outdated). Bibliography, however, is a *gold mine* for those seeking guidance on financing for board and care homes.

**Dallek, G., ed. *Insuring the Uninsured: Options for State Action*. Washington, DC: National Health Care Campaign, 1987. $25.00. Excellent review of Medicaid and indigent care program expansion, COBRA health insurance, state health insurance issues, and much more.

**Dallek, G., *et al*. *The Best Medicine: Organizing Local Health Care Campaigns*. Washington, DC: The Villers Foundation, 1984 (1988 *Supplement*). $7.00. How to change and liberalize Medicaid, indigent care, Hill-Burton, and other health programs. A bible for reform activists.

*Dalton, H., ed. *AIDS and the Law, A Guide for the Public*. New Haven and London: Yale University Press, 1987. $8.95. General PWA issues, especially legal rights and discrimination.

*Dean, D. *Doctors For the Poor: Increasing Physician Participation in Medicaid*. Chicago: National Clearinghouse for Legal Services, 1987. $10.50. Order no. 43,205.

*Deets, H. *Prescription for Action: A Guide to Community Health Reform*. Washington, DC: AARP, 1987. Free. Organizing at the local level to reform and expand health care.

**Deford, G. "Medicaid Liens, Recoveries, and Transfers of Assets After TEFRA" in *Clearinghouse Review* 18 (June 1984): 134. Chicago: National Clearinghouse for Legal Services. $6.00. A *must* for those planning to avoid Medicaid/welfare asset limits, or trying to preserve PWA assets and homes from later state recoupments of Medicaid-financed care.

**Department of Housing and Urban Development. *Programs of HUD*. Washington, DC: HUD, 1989. (Publication No. HUD-214-PA[16]). Free. Grants and loans to purchase, construct, renovate, expand, establish, equip, staff, and operate board and care homes. See discussions of rehabilitation loans under sec. 312, emergency shelter grants, loans to nonprofit sponsors of sec. 202 projects, sec. 221 (d), sec. 202, sec. 231, sec. 17 of U.S. Housing Act of 1937, sec. 232, congregate housing services, sec. 241, flexible subsidies, supportive housing demonstration grants, transitional housing grants, supportive housing demonstration program, and supplemental assistance for facilities to assist the homeless. This booklet also contains regional and local HUD office addresses and telephone numbers for further inquiries about these funding sources.

Department of Justice. *Memorandum Re: Application of Section 504 of the Rehabilitation Act to Persons With AIDS.* Chicago: National Clearinghouse for Legal Services, 1986. $5.25. Order no. 41,410.

*Desonia, R., and K. King. *State Programs of Assistance for the Medically Indigent.* Washington, DC: Intergovernmental Health Policy Project, George Washington University, 1985. For a basic understanding of the origins and bases of state General Medical Assistance/indigent care programs (such as those for non-Medicaid-type people). Dated, but a good starting point. Unfortunately out of print.

Desonia, R., and D. Lipson, eds. *Major Changes in State Medicaid and Indigent Care Programs* (annual editions, 1984–). Washington, DC: Intergovernmental Health Policy Project, George Washington University, 1984–1988. $25.00 per edition.

Disability Evaluation Under Social Security. Baltimore: Social Security Administration, 1986. Free. "Listing of Impairments" of disabling conditions, according to diagnostic group. Turgid, nearly incomprehensible prose in a highly stylized format, but this is how SSA operates. Unfortunately, this edition is not timely enough to incorporate AIDS data.

Dittmar, N. *Board and Care for Elderly and Mentally Disabled Populations.* Denver: Denver Research Institute, 1983.

*Dobkin, Leah. *The Board and Care System: A Regulatory Jungle.* Washington, DC: AARP, 1989. Free. How one state's (Maryland's) board and care home system operates and how it can be streamlined. Includes the "Model Act Regulating Board and Care Homes: Guidelines for States."

Dorn, S., J. Perkins, and R. Schwartz. "Maximizing Coverage for Medicaid Clients" in *Clearinghouse Review* 20 (1986): 441. Chicago: National Clearinghouse for Legal Services, 1986. $6.00.

Dowell, M. *State and Local Government Legal Responsibilities to Provide Medical Care for the Poor.* Chicago: National Clearinghouse for Legal Services, 1989. $25.00. Order no. 40,275.

**Eidson, T., ed. *The AIDS Caregiver's Handbook.* New York: St. Martin's, 1988. $10.95. *The* "how-to" manual for all *non*-eligibility advocacy, social work, volunteer, and other supportive roles.

Ellis, L., and R. Thewes. *Lifelink Life Counseling Workbook.* Washington, DC: Lifelink, 1988. Free. Typical local volunteer materials for assisting PWAs in applying for benefits.

Erdman, K., and S. Wolfe. *Poor Health Care for Poor Americans: A Ranking of State Medicaid Programs.* Washington, DC: Public Citizen Research Group, 1987.

*Eskin, R., and H. Grant. *Food Stamp Advocates Manual*. Chicago: National Clearinghouse for Legal Services, 1983. $6.00. Order no. 33,840B. Good introduction, but now slightly dated.

**Fraser, I. *Medicaid Options: State Opportunities and Strategies for Expanding Eligibility*. Chicago: American Hospital Association, 1987. Free.

**Freifeld, A. *The Right to Health Care: An Advocate's Guide to the Hill-Burton Uncompensated Care and Community Services Requirements*. Chicago: National Clearinghouse for Legal Services, 1986. $15.00. Order no. 41,900. The bible for working with Hill-Burton issues and cases.

**Fried, B., *et al*. *Health Care For All: Medicaid Expansion*. Washington, DC: National Health Care Campaign, 1987. $25.00. How to advocate for a state Medicaid program which will cover all of the poor disabled.

**Fried, Bruce, ed. *Representing Older Persons*. Chicago: National Clearinghouse for Legal Services, 1986. $15.00. Order no. 38,950. Eligibility for SSDI, SSI, Medicare, Medicaid, waivers/long-term care and much else—this is for the *disabled* as well as the aged. Comprehensive, but weak in setting forth state variations and procedural "how to's" in dealing with SSA/welfare offices. Very legalistic, and therefore tough going for nonlawyer advocates—this should be in every PWA benefits advocacy office.

*Fuchs, F. *Introduction to HUD-Subsidized Housing Programs*. Chicago: National Clearinghouse for Legal Services, 1984. $11.50. Order no. 33,843B. A good, thorough introduction to this complex set of programs, but slightly dated.

Gillett, R. *Foreclosure Prevention Programs Available to Homeowners With Governmentally Insured Mortgages*. Chicago: National Clearinghouse for Legal Services, 1985. $1.75. Order no. 40,251. Excerpted in this book.

**Greater Upstate Law Project. *Representing Disability Claimants Before the Social Security Administration—a Primer for New Advocates*. Chicago: National Clearinghouse for Legal Services, 1985. $12.00. Order no. 40,208.

Gong, V. *Understanding AIDS: A Comprehensive Guide*. New Brunswick: Rutgers University Press, 1985. $10.95.

Halahan, J., and J. Cohen. *Medicaid: The Trade-Off Between Cost Containment and Access to Care*. Washington, DC: Urban Institute, 1986.

Hall, C. *NAN Directory*. Washington, DC: National AIDS Network, 1988. Free to members. Listing of local AIDS service organizations.

Halleron, T., and J. Pisaneschi. *AIDS Information Resources Directory*. New York: American Foundation for AIDS Research, 1988. $39.95.

*Harmon, Carolyn. *Board and Care: A New Resource for Long Term Care*. Washington, DC: Center for the Study of Social Policy, 1982. $5.00. Another good introduction to the use of those facilities; this includes brief discussions of innovative programs in several states to finance upgrading and renovation.

Health Care Financing Administration, U.S. Department of Health and Human Services. *Health Insurance Manual*. Baltimore: Health Care Financing Administration. Medicare manual; available for public examination in SSA offices.

**Health Resources and Services Administration. "Project Grants for Renovation or Construction of Non-Acute Care Intermediate and Long-Term Care Facilities for Patients with Acquired Immune Deficiency Syndrome (AIDS)" in 54 *Federal Register* No. 89 (May 10, 1989; pp. 20205–20208). $1.40. This announcement was for fiscal 1989, but funding in subsequent years is expected to continue.

*Humphry, D. *Let Me Die Before I Wake*. Eugene, OR: The Hemlock Society, 1986. $11.50. Contains instructions on the actual methods (drug dosages) for a terminally ill person to accelerate the end.

**Intergovernmental Health Policy Project, George Washington University. *AIDS and Prescription Drug Therapy: Paying the Bill*. Pamphlet series, state by state. Washington, DC: IHPP, 1987. Slightly dated, but brief descriptions of state AZT, Medicaid, and General Medical Assistance programs are very helpful. Also available free from National Association of People With AIDS.

**James, P. *Guide for Social Security Disability Insurance Claims for HIV Disease—AIDS-ARC*. San Francisco: AIDS Benefits Counselors, 1988. $30.00 An *absolute must* for anyone who must apply or advocate for an SSDI/SSI "ARC-only" claim. *Very* good on how to document, write up, and assemble medical, psychological, and social data to produce a successful disability award. *Warning:* Forms and procedures are those of *California* state agencies, which handle disability claims processing for SSA under contract *there*. In other states SSA uses *those* states' disability agencies and *their* forms and procedures. Thus, this manual can only be generalized to SSDI/SSI claims in other states on *a substantive* basis.

*James, P., G. Wood, and A. Philipson. *AIDS-Related Condition (ARC) Social Security Disability Insurance Claims*. San Francisco: AIDS Legal Referral Panel, 1987. $20.00. An earlier, slightly less comprehensive, but still useful version of the above listed work.

*Jameson, Barbara. *Directory of Residential Care Facilities*. Richmond, Va.: National Association of Residential Care Facilities, 1988. Free. This not only lists state board and care home associations, it also contains listings of licensure officials and descriptions/enrollment forms for the inexpensive NARCF-sponsored Board and Care Home Administrator Certification Program courses, which are vital for licensure.

*Joe, T., et al. *Completing the Long Term Care Continuum*. Washington, DC: Center for the Study of Social Policy, 1988. $10.00. A survey of 7 states' SSP programs to finance board and care home costs of the needy aged and disabled.

Joe, T., et al. *Restructuring Medicaid*. Washington, DC: Center for the Study of Social Policy, 1984.

Joe, T., et al. *Wolves in Sheeps' Clothing: Administrative Streamlining or Benefit Cuts*. Washington, DC: Center for the Study of Social Policy, 1983. $5.00. Reagan administration attempts to cut the SSI program.

Kenesson, M., et al. *Medical Assistance Manual: Eligibility*. Baltimore: Health Care Financing Administration, U.S. Department of Health and Human Services, 1975–1980. Now somewhat dated, this is a good narrative explanation of the federal requirements and state choices in Medicaid eligibility policy. Out of print, but available for copying on request.

Kennedy, W. *New Hampshire Benefits Guide for Older Citizens*. Washington, DC: AARP, 1986. Free. Programs for aged apply to disabled persons too.

*Komlos-Hrobsky, P. *An Advocate's Guide to Home Care for the Elderly*. Chicago: National Clearinghouse for Legal Services, 1986. $15.00. Order no. 43,200.

Koop, C. *Surgeon General's Report on Acquired Immune Deficiency Syndrome*. Washington, DC: U.S. Department of Health and Human Services, 1987. Free.

Kopper, M., ed. *Elder Law Forum*. Periodical. Washington, DC: Legal Counsel for the Elderly, 1988–. Legislation, developments, and court cases about programs and issues concerning the aged and disabled.

Koyonagi, C. *Operation Help: A Mental Health Advocate's Guide to Medicaid*. Alexandria, Va.: National Mental Health Association, 1988. $25.00.

Laudicina, A. "Financing For AIDS Care" in *Journal of Ambulatory Care Management* 11 (May 1988): 55. Home, community, and hospice care is more appropriate—and nearly $4,000 cheaper per AIDS case—than hospitalization.

Laudicina, A. "States Move Ahead to Pay For Costs Related to AIDS" in *The Internist* 29 (Aug. 1988): 10. Outpatient AZT is not covered in Alabama, Arkansas, and Colorado. (Nor is it covered in Texas and Wyoming.)

**Legal Counsel for the Elderly. *Decision-Making, Incapacity, and the Elderly*. Washington, DC: Legal Counsel for the Elderly, 1987. $29.95.

*Legal Counsel for the Elderly. *Disability (Social Security and SSI Programs)*. Washington, DC: Legal Counsel for the Elderly, 1984. $3.95. Overview and questions and answers on disability determination rules and procedures.

*Legal Counsel for the Elderly. *Elderly Law Manual*. Washington, DC: Legal Counsel for the Elderly, 1985. $19.95. Desk reference manual, especially on benefits program eligibility, written in style suitable for volunteers.

**Legal Counsel for the Elderly. *Food Stamps Training Module*. Washington, DC: Legal Counsel for the Elderly, 1989. $7.00. Contains model eligibility examples for learning computations, as well as a good review of program rules.

**Legal Counsel for the Elderly. *Lay Advocacy Handbook*. Washington, DC: Legal Counsel for the Elderly, 1988. $3.95. How to set up and run a non-attorney volunteer program in the area of public benefits counseling and advocacy.

Legal Counsel for the Elderly. *Medicare: Obtaining Your Full Benefits*. Washington, DC: Legal Counsel for the Elderly, 1984.

**Legal Counsel for the Elderly. *Public Benefits Checklist*. Washington, DC: Legal Counsel for the Elderly, 1986. $2.95. Quick way to review and assess eligibility for many benefits programs; how to apply; ideal for training benefits advocate volunteers.

**Leonard, M., ed. *Clearinghouse Review*. Periodical. Chicago: National Clearinghouse for Legal Services. $75.00/year. *The* periodical devoted to advocacy for the poor disabled and others, especially for public benefits. Lawyerly, but indispensable to any high-volume advocacy effort.

*Leukfeld, C., and M. Fimbres, eds. *Responding to AIDS*. Silver Spring, Md: National Association of Social Workers, 1987. $9.95. Non-eligibility social work with PWAs.

Lingle, V., and M. Wood. *How To Find Information About AIDS*. New York: Harrington Park Press, 1988. $6.95. A good bibliography on AIDS in general, but skimpy on benefits issues.

Low Income Home Energy Assistance Program: Report to Congress for Fiscal Year 1987. Washington, DC: Family Support Administration, HHS, 1988. Free.

Lybarger, B., and N. Onerheim. *An Advocate's Guide to Surviving the SSI System*. Boston: Massachusetts Poverty Law Center, 1985.

McCormack, T. *Applying for Medicaid*. Flyer. Washington, DC: Whitman-Walker Clinic, 1985. Typical "how to" material on local Medicaid eligibility, used by local AIDS service group.

McCormack, T. *Eligibility for Social Security Disability, Supplemental Security Income (SSI), Welfare, Food Stamps and Housing Help*. Pamphlet. Washington, DC: Whitman-Walker Clinic, 1985. Programs, rules, and examples of eligibility in these programs; used by local AIDS service group. Now slightly dated.

McCormack, T. *Using Supplemental Security Income (SSI) and DC Funds To Help Operate Community Residence Facilities*. Washington, DC: Whitman-Walker Clinic, 1984. Discussion paper on use of local SSP for board and care homes to fund group housing services for PWAs.

Martelli, L., *et al. When Someone You Know Has AIDS: A Practical Guide*. New York: Crown Publishers, 1987. $9.95. Fear, grief, finances, and legal and medical issues. Very thin on public benefit eligibility, however.

Medicaid Services State By State. Baltimore, MD: Health Care Financing Administration, U.S. Department of Health and Human Services. Free.

**Medicare and Medicaid Guide*. Multi-volume legal looseleaf service. Chicago: Commerce Clearing House, Inc., 1966–. Several hundred dollars annual subscription. Mind-boggling in its historical depth, comprehensiveness, complexity, and cost, this is a "must" for legal advocates for PWA Medicaid benefits. Nonlawyers proceed with caution—this is very legalistic.

Medicare and Medicaid: There Is a Difference! South Deerfield, Mass: Channing L. Bete, 1986. Pamphlet. Free. Good pamphlet simply explaining programs; available at SSA offices.

Miller-Reimer, C., ed. *Accessing Illinois Department of Public Aid and Social Security Administration Entitlements For Persons With Acquired Immune Deficiency Syndrome*. Chicago: Howard Brown Memorial Clinic, 1988. One of the few locally produced manuals for PWA benefits advocates. Comprehensive coverage of local SSDI, SSI, SSP, GA, AFDC, Medicaid, Food Stamps, and General Medical Assistance. Very useful for *other* Illinois advocacy organizations but inapplicable in other states. A helpful model for preparation of other locality-specific PWA benefits advocacy handbooks.

**Milstein, B., B. Pepper, and L. Rubenstein "The Fair Housing Amendments Act of 1988: What It Means for People with Mental Disabilities" in *Clearinghouse Review* 23 (June 1989):128. Chicago: National Clearinghouse For Legal Services, 1989. $6.00. It means that states, localities, and neighborhood groups are now barred from blocking group homes for the disabled under the guise of zoning and similar procedures.

**Mishkin, B. *A Matter of Choice: Planning Ahead for Health Care Decisions.* Washington, DC: AARP, 1986. Free. The right to decide on health care, guardianship, court orders, living wills, durable powers of attorney, and dying.

Moffatt, B. *When Someone You Love Has AIDS: A Book of Hope For Family and Friends.* Santa Monica: IBS Press, 1986. $9.95. Good companion volume to the above listing.

*Moffatt, B., et al. *AIDS: A Self Care Manual.* Santa Monica: IBS Press, 1987. $12.95. Helpful for benefits advocates and PWAs in covering noneligibility care and life issues.

Monette, Paul. *On Borrowed Time: An AIDS Memoir.* San Diego: Harcourt, Brace, Jovanovich, 1987. What it's like for PWA, lover, and family—from start to finish.

*Moses, S. *Medicaid Estate Recoveries.* Seattle: Department of Health and Human Services, 1988. Free. How thousands with large assets still manage to receive free Medicaid care.

Mullen, J., and C. Schneider. *Medicaid Cutbacks: A Handbook for Beneficiary Advocates.* Chicago: National Clearinghouse for Legal Services, 1976.

*National Gay Rights Advocates. *AIDS and Your Legal Rights.* Pamphlet. San Francisco: NGRA, 1988. Good general rundown of PWA rights, including brief discussion of entitlements.

*National Health Law Program. *An Advocate's Guide to the Medically Needy Program.* Los Angeles: National Health Law Program, 1985. How to advocate for a state "medically needy spend down" program, and then how to work with it after its adoption.

*National Health Law Program. "Health Benefits: How the System Is Responding to AIDS" in *Clearinghouse Review* 22 (Dec. 1988): 724. Chicago: National Clearinghouse for Legal Services. $6.00. Good summary of where we were in health coverage programs for PWAs as of late 1988.

*National Health Law Program. *Legal Rights to Health Care For Persons With AIDS.* Pamphlet. Los Angeles: NHLP, 1988. Free. Similar to above NGRA pamphlet.

O'Connor, T. *Living With AIDS: Reaching Out.* San Francisco: Corwin Publications, 1986. Touches only briefly on public benefits.

O'Sullivan, J. *Medicaid: Legislative History, Program Description, and Major Issues.* Washington, DC: Congressional Research Service, 1984. Free.

Pascal, A. "The Cost of Treating AIDS Under Medicaid: 1986–1991." Santa Monica: Rand Corporation, 1987. It will be a lot—billions and billions of dollars.

**Pepper, B. "The Impact of the Fair Housing Amendments on Land Use Regulations Affecting People with Disabilities." Washington, DC: Mental Health

Law Project, 1989. Free. (Flyer) How federal law now effectively outlaws state and local zoning, licensure, density, use permit, variance, neighborhood notification/consent or building permit laws, rules and procedures as ways to discriminatorily block group homes for the disabled.

Perkins, J. "ERISA Preemption Affecting Indigent Health Care Coverage" in *Clearinghouse Review* 20 (April 1987): 1506. Chicago: National Clearinghouse for Legal Services. $6.00.

Perkins, J., and R. Boyle. "AIDS and Poverty: Dual Barriers to Health Care" in *Clearinghouse Review* 19 (March 1986): 1283. Chicago: National Clearinghouse for Legal Services. $6.00.

**Perkins, J., and J. Waxman. "The COBRA Continuation Option: Questions and Answers" in *Clearinghouse Review* 21 (April 1988): 1315. Chicago: National Clearinghouse for Legal Services. $6.00. Essential for advocates in handling COBRA health insurance extensions/conversions for PWAs leaving employment.

*Ponce, E. *Characteristics of State Assistance Programs for SSI Recipients, January, 1989.* Baltimore: Social Security Administration, 1989. Published annually. Free. Basic data SSA gathers on SSPs, 1616 and 1634 status of states, Emergency Assistance, and General Assistance. To be used with caution: data, particularly on SSP levels, is 6 to 12 months old by yearly publication date.

**Program Operations Manual Systems (POMS).* Baltimore: Social Security Administration. SSA's manual on SSDI, SSI, SSPs, disability determination, Medicare, Medicaid, and much else. Benefits advocates need to review this for at least a few hours. (*Serious* study would take a lifetime!) Available for viewing at SSA offices.

Regan, J., and Legal Counsel for the Elderly. *Your Legal Rights in Later Life.* Glenview, IL: Scott, Foresman, and Company, 1989. $9.95. Sketchy review of SSDI, SSI, VA, Medicare, and Medicaid eligibility.

**Reisacher, S. "Quality of Care: Operation and Management Issues" in M. Moon, G. Gaberlavage, and S. Newman, eds. *Preserving Independence, Supporting Needs: The Role of Board and Care Homes.* Washington, DC: AARP, 1989. Free.

**Reschovsky, J. "Present and Future Roles of HUD Programs in Board and Care Financing" in M. Moon, G. Gaberlavage, and S. Newman, eds. *Preserving Independence, Supporting Needs: The Role of Board and Care Homes.* Washington, DC: AARP, 1989. Free.

Roper, W. "From the Health Care Financing Administration" in *Journal of the American Medical Association* 258 (Dec. 1987): 3489. Due to 2-year waiting period for Medicare, few PWAs survive long enough to generate Medicare-covered expenses; but over 40% of PWAs receive at least some Medicaid coverage.

Rowe, M., and C. Ryan. "Comparing State-Only Expenditures for AIDS" in *American Journal of Public Health* 78 (April, 1988): 424.

*Schatz, B. *Access to AIDS-Related Drugs Under Medicaid: A Fifty-State Analysis.* San Francisco: National Gay Rights Advocates, 1989. $12.95. Excerpted in this book.

**Scherzer, M. "Insurance and AIDS-Related Issues" in *AIDS Practice Manual: A Legal and Educational Guide*. San Francisco: National Gay Rights Advocates, 1988. $35.00. Important on COBRA and other insurance-related matters of concern to PWAs.

**Schuster, M. *Disability Practice Manual* (and *1986–1987* and *1988–1989 Supplements*). Washington, DC: Legal Counsel for the Elderly, 1985, 1986. $45.00. Very legalistic manual about SSDI/SSI eligibility—especially disability determination rules, procedures, issues, and court cases. Especially good in discussing the intricate, multi-layered SSA disability case processing system and the truly arcane and Byzantine reconsideration/appeals/redetermination procedures. This book is an absolute necessity for those advocates (especially lawyers) handling difficult disability determination cases and appeals. Overwhelming to the lay advocate, the issues it covers are nearly incomprehensible to anyone but lifetime attorney specialists.

Schwartz, R. *An Advocate's Guide to the Medicaid Program*. Chicago: National Clearinghouse for Legal Services, 1985. $8.00. A restatement of federal Medicaid regulations and law—especially eligibility.

Shilts, R. *And the Band Played On: Politics, People, and the AIDS Epidemic*. New York: Viking-Penguin, 1987. How AIDS appeared and spread, and how the system slowly responded.

*Shuey, M. "The VA Improved Pension: What It Means for SSI and Medicaid Recipients" in *Clearinghouse Review* 19 (Aug./Sept. 1985): 463. Chicago: National Clearinghouse for Legal Services. $6.00. The VA doesn't count SSI, AFDC, and welfare income for its pension, but those programs (and Medicaid) *do* count VA pensions (except the "aid and attendance" increment).

**Sieradzki, M. *Buddy Programs*. Washington, DC: National AIDS Network, 1988. Free to members. How to set up and run volunteer peer support programs for people with HIV disease. Focuses on noneligibility social services.

Simpson, D. *Case Management in Long Term Care Programs*. Washington, DC: Center for the Study of Social Policy, 1982.

**Skala, Ken. *American Guidance for Those Over 60*. Falls Church, Va: Sharff Publications, 1989. $12.95. Parallels this text in some ways, but Skala focuses more on needs and programs for the middle-class elderly—not the poor disabled. Sketchy on eligibility for needs-based programs.

Skalnick, B., and P. Warrick. *The Right Place at the Right Time: A Guide to Long Term Care Choices*. Washington, DC: AARP, 1985. Free.

Smith, S. "Reducing the AIDS Bill" in *Governing* 2 (Feb. 1989): 52. Summary of costs of AIDS in hospital care, and a good review of state and local initiatives in alternatives to hospitalization, such as "2176" home and community-based services waivers and related programs.

**Social Security Administration. "Supplemental Security Income for the Aged, Blind, and Disabled. Presumptive Disability and Presumptive Blindness; Categories of Impairments—AIDS" in 53 *Federal Register* 26 (pp. 3739–3742) (February 9, 1988). Washington, DC: Office of the Federal Register, 1988. Can be

photocopied for less than $1.00 at any good legal library. Current SSDI/SSI
disability standards for AIDS, ARC, and "presumptive disability" determinations.
Contains list of "qualifying" opportunistic infections. See especially the preamble
material, since only it (and, unfortunately, *not the regulation's text itself*)
addresses exact procedures and standards for securing "presumptive eligibility"
under SSI for PWAs.

Social Security Bulletin. Baltimore: Social Security Administration. Periodical. SSA
publication of program developments and assorted data.

Social Security Forum. Periodical. Pearl River, N.Y.: National Organization of
Social Security Claimants' Representatives. A disability law advocate's
clearinghouse on SSDI and SSI.

Social Security Handbook. Baltimore: Social Security Administration, 1986. Useful
basic SSDI, SSI, and Medicare program information.

*_____. *State Plans*. U.S. Department of Health and Human Services, 1966–1989.
Unpublished, but open to public viewing and selective photocopying at central
office and 10 regional offices. Difficult in format and legalistic, these loose-leaf-
bindered sheets set forth each state's eligibility and coverage rules, as purported to
be currently in force, for the Medicaid, AFDC, Emergency Assistance, Social
Services (Title XX), SSP, Energy Assistance, and other programs. Not for the
fainthearted.

Stefl, M. *Helping Mentally Ill Homeless People: A Manual for Shelter Workers*.
Washington, DC: American Public Health Association, 1989. $10.00. Sketchy on
benefits eligibility, but good on general social work.

**Steinberg, Susan. *How To Prepare and Conduct a Social Security Disability
Hearing*. Chicago: National Clearinghouse for Legal Services, 1985. $10.50.
Order no. 40,700.

**Stiehl, W. J., *Baxter v. Belleview* (Cause No. 89-3354, U.S.D.C., S.D., ILL.,
August 25, 1989), 1989 WESTLAW 10196, 720 Federal Supplement 720.
(Available in any good law library.) Injunction of federal district court outlawing a
city's denial of zoning clearance for a PWA group home under the Fair Housing
Amendments Act of 1988.

Stone, R., R. Newcomer, and M. Saunders. *Descriptive Analysis of Board and Care
Policy in the Fifty States*. San Francisco: University of California at San Francisco,
Aging Health Policy Center, 1982. (Address: Post Office Box 0834, San
Francisco, CA 94143-0834.) Review of *state* programs to fund the establishment
and improvement of board and care homes and to train staff.

Sulveta, M., and K. Swartz. *The Uninsured and Uncompensated Care*. Washington,
DC: Urban Institute, 1986.

**Sweeney, E. *Supplemental Security Income (SSI): Income, Resources and
Procedural Issues*. Los Angeles: National Senior Citizens' Law Center, 1989.
Most recent update on SSI program changes and developments.

**Tallon, J., *et al*. *Health Policy Agenda for the American People: Medicaid
Reform*. Materials package. Chicago: American Medical Association, 1989. Free.
Why Medicaid doesn't cover everyone who needs it, and a broad plan to reform it.

**Torda, P. *The Medicare Catastrophic Protection Act* and *Qualified Medicare Buy-In ("QMB")*. Pamphlets and flyers. Washington, DC: The Villers Foundation, 1988. Free. How Medicare has changed and ways in which Medicaid can also be improved under new federal legislation. Useful in understanding how to advocate effectively for state improvements.

Torrey, E., S. Wolfe, and L. Flynn. *Care of the Seriously Mentally Ill.* Washington, DC: Public Citizen Health Research Group, 1986. Discussion of state mental health/public mental hospital programs.

Von Behren, L., ed. *Joint Conference on Law and Aging (October 13–15, 1988).* Proceedings. Washington, DC: Legal Counsel for the Elderly, 1988. Free. Developments in programs and advocacy for the aged and disabled, especially in benefits eligibility.

*Warren, A., and D. Pritchett. *Paying More, Getting Less: How U.S. Health Care Measures Up.* Washington, DC: National Health Care Campaign, 1988. The United States is the only industrialized country without national health care, yet it spends more money than others.

*Wetch, P., *et al. Independence Through Interdependence.* Boston: Massachusetts Department of Elder Affairs, 1984. Free. How to plan, set up, and run a "congregate living facility"; this is a broad designation for board and care homes and related projects. Good on planning, building, site selection, tenant placement, and social arrangement issues, but very weak on licensure as board and care home, use for disabled as opposed to aged, and applicability of SSP financing/coverage/placement.

Whitman-Walker Clinic. *Legal Answers About AIDS.* Pamphlet. Washington, DC: WWC, 1988.

**Wulsin, L. "Adopting a Medically Needy Program" in *Clearinghouse Review* 18 (Dec. 1984): 841. Chicago: National Clearinghouse for Legal Services. $6.00. Technical information necessary to advocate for adding a "medically needy spend down" to a state Medicaid program.

**Zimmerman, D. *2176 Waivers.* Washington, DC: National AIDS Network, 1988. $15.00. What are these Medicaid waivers? And how to advocate for one in your state.

The following multi-volume sets of the *Code of Federal Regulations* should be available in any good law library. They can also be purchased from the U.S. Government Printing Office, Washington, DC 20001, (202) 783–3238.

7 C.F.R. 271–. Food Stamp regulations.

7 C.F.R. 1872, 17, 1900, 1944.34, 1951.213, 1951.312, 1951.313, 1951.314, 1955. FMHA Mortgage delinquency regulations.

**20 C.F.R. 404.1–.2127. Social Security Disability Insurance (SSDI) regulations.

**20 C.F.R. 216–. Supplemental Security Income (SSI) regulations.

24 C.F.R. 203. FHA and HUD mortgage delinquency regulations.

24 C.F.R. 900–. Federal housing program regulations.

38 C.F.R. _____. Department of Veterans Affairs program regulations.

38 C.F.R. 36.4301–4355. VA mortgage delinquency regulations.

42 C.F.R. 124. Hill-Burton program regulations.

42 C.F.R. 405–429. Medicare regulations.

42 C.F.R. 430–499. Medicaid regulations.

45 C.F.R. _____. AFDC and Emergency Assistance regulations.

Index